Nursing ethics

Nursing ethics

A principle-based approach

Steven D. Edwards

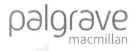

Published by
PALGRAVE MACMILLAN
Houndmills, Basingstoke, Hampshire RG21 6XS and
175 Fifth Avenue, New York, N.Y. 10010
Companies and representatives throughout the world

PALGRAVE MACMILLAN is the global academic imprint of the Palgrave
Macmillan division of St. Martin's Press, LLC and of Palgrave Macmillan Ltd.
Macmillan® is a registered trademark in the United States, United Kingdom
and other countries. Palgrave is a registered trademark in the European
Union and other countries.

ISBN 0–333–61590–5

This book is printed on paper suitable for recycling and
made from fully managed and sustained forest sources.

A catalogue record for this book is available from the British Library.

Transferred to digital printing 2002

Printed and bound in Great Britain by
Antony Rowe Limited, Chippenham and Eastbourne

Contents

Preface

I have tried to produce a degree-level text in nursing ethics, but one which will be of use to nursing diploma students, to those studying nursing ethics at postgraduate level, and to registered nurses who are undertaking short courses in nursing ethics. I became aware of the need for such a text between 1991 and 1993. During this period I was required to write and to teach a number of courses in nursing ethics at varying levels. There are, of course, several books on nursing ethics, but none seemed to be at just the right level for the needs of the students I taught. Although many students found Melia (1989) and Chadwick and Tadd (1992) extremely useful introductions to the subject, these texts seemed not to provide material beyond diploma level.

The most thorough treatment of health care ethics that I am aware of is Beauchamp and Childress's *Principles of Biomedical Ethics* (1989, 1994). It is no understatement to reveal that this book changed my whole outlook on nursing ethics and this is evident throughout the following text. The students I taught, however, did not seem to find Beauchamp and Childress user-friendly; they found it too dense and too medically orientated. Hence, it has been my intention to provide a text which approximates the systematicity of Beauchamp and Childress's work, but which is more accessible to students of nursing ethics.

When I trained as a nurse, the curriculum included no ethics whatsoever. Yet, the moral problems encountered during my time in nursing drove me to study philosophy at undergraduate level. It soon became apparent that, at that time (the mid-eighties), the subject matter of ethics courses made no mention of the kinds of moral problems which arise in nursing practice. Further, I came to realise that the problem of moral knowledge was merely a part of a larger problem of knowledge in general.

This led me into the problem of philosophical relativism and far away from applied ethics.

A peculiar chain of events resulted in my obtaining a post which involved nothing other than teaching nursing ethics. This gave me the opportunity to re-examine the moral problems which I had faced as a nurse many years earlier, and this book forms part of that ongoing examination.

I have benefited greatly over the years from discussion of moral matters with very many people. But I would like to acknowledge particular debts of gratitude to the 1991 intake of nursing students at Buckinghamshire College of Higher Education, to Ed Lepper and to Simon Woods.

Swansea   STEVEN D. EDWARDS

Introduction

Crudely, this book is an attempt to apply to nursing ethics the approach to bioethics which is set out by Beauchamp and Childress in their *Principles of Biomedical Ethics* (1989, 1994). It should be stressed, though, that there are differences between the claims set out by Beauchamp and Childress and claims made in this book. Further, at least one of these differences is quite fundamental in that in their book they claim to reject any hierarchical ordering of principles (1989, p. 125), but in the present text it is tentatively claimed that the principle of respect for autonomy is 'weightier', so to speak, than other moral principles.

It should be said in introduction to what follows that no attempt has been made to discuss or describe all the types of moral problems which nurses are likely to encounter during the course of their practice; any such attempt is doomed to failure. Instead, what has been done is to try to set out a general approach which can then be applied to very many of the types of moral problems which arise in nursing practice. In particular, the approach set out here applies to moral problems arising from attempts to care for competent clients. (Throughout the book, the term 'client' is employed in preference to 'patient', but only on the grounds that 'client' is marginally less objectionable than 'patient'.)

Chapter 1 begins with an attempt to offer an outline of some of the ways in which people understand the term 'ethics'; this is followed by arguments in support of the claim that nurses should study ethics, and the outline of a strategy to aid recognition of moral issues. This should enable the reader to 'climb on', so to speak, to the framework for moral reasoning set out in Chapters 2 and 3.

In Chapter 2, I have tried to explain and describe the nature of the four levels of Beauchamp and Childress's framework,

1

and to explain the relations between these. More detailed accounts of the four level-three moral principles to be recruited are provided in Chapter 3; and justification for the weight accorded to the principle of respect for autonomy is, in part, provided in this chapter.

Chapter 4 focuses on the application of the principles. It is proposed that the onus of justification lies with those who attempt to override the competent, autonomous decisions of clients. As will be evident to readers, the application of this position to the moral problems arising from the care of persons with suicidal intentions causes great problems and the position arrived at is, it seems, supported by reason but conflicts with the emotions. This very conflict takes us to the heart of a challenge to the principle-based approach from the perspective of a care-based approach to ethics.

In Chapter 5, the nature of the challenge to the principle-based line from the care-based perspective is set out. It is concluded that a position in which principles are applied in a caring way is the most favourable, and arguments are provided against a purely care-based line.

The concluding chapter of the book is perhaps the most abstract. It attempts to show how the principles operant in the principle-based approach can help to structure thought concerning matters within nursing ethics, and to foster clearer analysis and thinking in relation to such matters. It is the author's view that the concluding remarks offered in this chapter carry serious implications for the nursing profession. They are intended to provoke further discussion of the issues raised in Chapter 6.

1 *Preliminary matters*

In this first chapter, an attempt is made to provide the reader with a rough, but adequate, understanding of the term 'ethics'. Three ways of employing the term are identified. Following this, the question of why nurses should study ethics at all is addressed. In the final section of the chapter, a strategy to aid the identification of moral issues in nursing is attempted.

What is ethics?

Crudely, ethics may be described as the enquiry into certain situations and into the language employed to describe them. This definition may be of limited help, however, since it does not enable us to distinguish those situations which have an ethical aspect, from those which do not. Shortly, we will attempt to say how situations with an ethical aspect can be identified, but before this it will prove useful to set out a rough distinction between three senses of the term 'ethics' (or, equivalently, 'morals'). For present purposes, we can follow the convention of regarding the terms 'ethics' and 'morals' as synonyms (see, for example, Singer, 1979, p. 1, 1991, p. v; Thompson, Melia and Boyd, 1988, p. 2; Seedhouse, 1988, p. 18).

Personal ethics

The first sense of the term 'ethics' to be mentioned here concerns its use in the personal sense. When invited to offer a definition of ethics, many students understand the term in this fashion. Ethics in the personal sense, they suggest, refers to the beliefs which individuals hold about ethical issues – with regard to the way people ought to act and so on. Such beliefs stem from the (usually) informal moral education received from various sources: parents, schoolteachers, religious figures and the media. These sources influence the views of persons with

3

regard to moral matters and such views standardly inform the intuitive judgements voiced in relation to ethical issues.

People normally have opinions on ethical issues whether or not they have formally studied ethics. Someone may claim that it is wrong to abuse children or to kill animals for sport, for example. Such personal beliefs may be the result of deliberation by the persons concerned, in which case it could be expected that they are able to supply reasons in support of their views: for example, it is wrong to kill animals for sport because it is wrong to kill humans for sport, and humans are animals. A person who argues against killing animals in this way may assume there to be no distinction in morality between killing humans and killing non-human animals.

Alternatively, a person might not be able to provide any reasons in support of their view; such a person may say simply that they know it is wrong to kill animals for sport without being able to say just why it is wrong. In everyday arguments about moral issues, people frequently appeal to their moral intuitions: they claim simply to know that some courses of action are wrong even though they cannot say why. Child abuse may present a useful example here. Most people find this practice morally abhorrent, and, generally, do not believe that any reasons are required in support of such a view: it is wrong to abuse children and that's that.

It seems plausible to claim that almost all people, able to express a view, hold positions on many situations with an ethical aspect. These positions reflect their own ethics: their own views of what is right and what is wrong.

Group ethics

A second sense of the term 'ethics' – one of particular relevance to members of the nursing profession – involves reference to the ethics of a group. These may be formal statements of standards of behaviour which members are expected to act in accordance with. Such a group might be a professional group such as nurses, footballers or medical staff, or a religious group – we could think of the Ten Commandments in this context.

Nurses comprise a useful example of a professional group which has proposed various codes of ethics. For example, the

American Nurses Association in 1976 and 1985 set out a Code of Ethics which identified the standards of behaviour expected of its members (see Benjamin and Curtis, 1986, pp. 179–81), and the equivalent body in the UK, the United Kingdom Central Council for Nursing, Midwifery and Health Visiting (UKCC) has set out a Code of Conduct (UKCC, 1992) which performs a similar function. Since there is a plethora of literature concerning codes of conduct for nurses, this second sense of the term 'ethics' will not be pursued for now. (For further information on codes of conduct, see, for example, Chadwick and Tadd, 1992, ch. 1; Burnard and Chapman, 1988; Benjamin and Curtis, 1986, ch. 1.)

Philosophical ethics

The third, and last, sense of the term 'ethics' to be identified here refers to ethics as a more formal and academic enterprise, which we can usefully describe as philosophical ethics. Within this, we can distinguish three general types of activity.

1. The development of *ethical theories* which attempt to set out prescriptions for morally right action. This may be done by attempting to show that acts which accord with certain criteria are morally preferable to other acts. Such criteria comprise a set of justifications for particular actions, or types of actions. Hence, a particular act, A (say, telling the truth), may be adjudged to be morally preferable to a different act, B (say, lying), since A accords with the criteria proposed in the theory and B does not. Two examples of theories devised in this way are Utilitarianism (for example Mill, 1863) and Kant's duty-based moral theory (Kant, 1785). Crudely, according to the Utilitarian, acts are right in so far as they maximise benefits or minimise harms. And, equally crudely, according to Kant, the rightness or wrongness of an act depends upon the motives of the actor.

    We will be looking at these two moral theories in greater detail in the next chapter. They are given here as examples of one of the kinds of activities which constitute philosophical ethics. It should be added that the approach to ethics to be set out in the present volume may amount to a theory in the sense under discussion here, for, as will be seen, the approach attempts to identify justifications for acting in one way rather than in others.

2. A second component of philosophical ethics consists in the *analytical enterprise* of examining moral claims, concepts and theories. This involves, for example, searching for inconsistency in moral argument and unclarity in moral concepts. This enterprise differs from the first activity discussed above in that it does not itself involve the proposal of substantive claims concerning what constitutes right or wrong action.

    We will be required to engage in philosophical ethics in this second sense. As will be seen, it is important to be especially clear when it comes to definitions of key terms and principles. Attention to clarity reduces the risk of misunderstanding and fosters a rigorous approach to the subject matter.

3. The third kind of activity describable under the rubric of philosophical ethics is so-called *metaethics*. This involves an examination of the language of morals itself. From the perspective of metaethics one asks questions such as: Can there be any moral facts? Is moral language meaningful? This differs from the second type of philosophical ethics in the sense that it queries the whole nature and language of morals.

    Perhaps unfortunately, we will not be engaged in any metaethical tasks in this book. It will simply be presumed – not unreasonably – that moral language is meaningful. Nor will the question of whether there can be moral facts be addressed (those interested may find Raphael [1981] a useful introduction). It is not being presumed that there are such facts, rather, it is supposed here that that question is less relevant to our concerns than the matters to be investigated during the course of this book.

This, then, completes a description of three senses of the term 'ethics'. Before moving on to the next section, it may be worth pausing briefly to consider the relations between these three kinds of activity, and also to consider their relevance to members of the nursing profession.

It is clear that the majority of nurses hold ethical views; hence they have an ethics in the first sense of the term described above. It is also clear that these beliefs about moral matters which individual nurses hold carry implications for the way certain moral problems encountered in professional practice will be viewed. For example, nurses who believe homosexual relationships to be wrong may find it difficult to deal with clients who are homosexual (see, for example, Viens, 1990 for a discussion of this issue).

Furthermore, a nurse who believes homosexual activities to be morally wrong, might find that this particular moral view conflicts with certain clauses in the UKCC Code of Conduct (for example, clause 7, 1992). Such a nurse would then experience a conflict between her personal ethics and the standards of behaviour expected of nurses by nurses themselves – since the UKCC Code is compiled by members of the nursing profession. It is evident, then, that courses of action which accord with one's personal ethical beliefs can conflict with courses of action required by the code of ethics (or conduct) recommended by one's professional body.

Engaging in some philosophical ethics can help to expose the source of such conflicts; this can be done by analysing and making explicit the moral principles which clash in such situations. Hopefully, the reader will be better able to undertake such analysis of moral conflicts after reading this book. For now, though, we move on to consider just why nurses should study ethics.

Why should nurses study ethics?

Ethical problems are frequently faced in our day-to-day lives. Suppose a person asks us for money for food. The situation may be thought to have an ethical aspect since one could benefit the person by giving some money; and one might be said to cause harm by omitting to give money. Or, suppose one sees an appeal in a newspaper which points out that £10 can save someone's sight, or maintain the life of a person in an extremely poor country (if only for a month). Should one send a donation? There are countless other, more mundane, examples of moral problems encountered on a regular basis: should one tell one's friend the horrible truth about his new haircut? should one try to avoid paying the bill at a restaurant? and so on. Clearly, we are capable of arriving at decisions concerning moral matters and can do so without doing a course in ethics. So why should nurses study ethics?

Below are some considerations which seem to be extremely relevant, and which help to support the claim that the moral intuition acquired and relied upon in ordinary everyday circumstances is of limited use in the health care setting. It is of limited use because the health care situation is different in many ways from the ordinary, everyday situations which we experience as part of our ordinary lives (see also Hussey, 1990).

- First, it is true to say that as a nurse one is faced with many more ethical problems than most ordinary members of the community have to face. In certain occupations it is possible to drift along happily without ever facing a serious moral dilemma. The sheer quantity of moral problems faced in the health care setting differs greatly from the quantity of moral problems one faces, generally speaking, in ordinary life. So, the moral context within which every day moral intuition is developed differs from the health care setting at least in the respect that in nursing practice the number of moral problems faced by nurses is significantly greater than is encountered by many people in many other types of occupations.
- Second, in our normal dealings with people on a day-to-day basis, we find people in their normal state – at home, in the pub or in the shop. They are in familiar surroundings with people they know, and they are in a situation in which they feel comfortable. (Of course this cannot be said of all people in the UK, but it can be said of a great many.) Clearly, none of this is true when clients are in hospital or when they or their close relatives are seriously ill. Clients may be extremely anxious, feel insecure, or perhaps even be unconscious (Hussey, 1990, p. 1377). So the usual, conventional setting within which we make moral decisions can again be seen to be radically different from the health care setting.
- Third, it may be the case that as a nurse one comes into contact with people who have had a different kind of moral

education, and so have developed different ways of respond-ing to moral problems. Consider, here, people from different ethnic backgrounds or people with different religious or pol-itical views. Many people do not have any prolonged contact with others who have had a radically different moral educa-tion than themselves. So, again, it can be seen to be the case that moral decision-making in nursing practice may differ from moral decision-making in ordinary circumstances. This is so because the nurse needs to take into account the per-spective of the person who has a different moral outlook than he or she. It may be added that the nurse is, in fact, required to do this by the UKCC Code (UKCC, 1992).

In ordinary, everyday life many people consider their own moral intuition to be unfailingly correct. For such people, moral conflicts do not arise. They simply assume that any moral views which diverge from the ones they themselves endorse must be wrong. But such an attitude is unsupport-able. It is necessary to consider at least the possibility that other moral views may be correct before it is possible to make any kind of adjudication between conflicting moral claims. It is not enough just to assert one's own moral views without considering other perspectives, and it is especially important for health care professionals to recognise this.

- Fourth, the availability of certain types of medical technology – for example, so-called life support machines – again makes the situation in the health care setting radically different from the normal context within which moral decisions are made. The point here is that in the health care setting the nurse will encounter moral dilemmas of a type which he or she will not have encountered previously in ordinary every-day life (Wright, 1993). Again, this indicates that the moral intuition developed in ordinary life is unlikely to be adequate to cope with the complex moral problems which arise in the health care context.

These last four points alone seem enough to support the claim that nurses should study ethics. It does seem plausible that the moral intuition developed and relied upon in normal circum-stances may be inadequate to cope with the quantity and the complexity of moral issues encountered in the health care setting. But there is a further, quite, general point which needs to be made.

Nurse education is changing rapidly – as, indeed, is the whole context of health care provision. One of the aims of this change is that nursing should be regarded as more of a profession than it has been hitherto. Part of the drive towards this recognition involves a degree of reflection upon the nature of nursing practice (Schon, 1987). This is why nurse education diplomas and degrees include nursing theory, and other disciplines which were not part of nurse education as it used to be. In studying ethics more formally, nurses are compelled to reflect upon moral decisions they have made (or may have to make in the future). The view is that reflection upon decisions made in practice makes for better nurses. Ethics is a subject which is particularly well suited to this aspect of nurse education. Most nurses are able to recount at least one ethical problem they have encountered in which they were unsure about the decision they made.

Perhaps unfortunately, studying ethics does not provide one with ready answers to the moral problems nurses face in their daily routine. What it does do is enable them to recognise moral problems, to have the conceptual equipment (common distinctions, knowledge of moral principles, and types of ethical theory) which can aid clear thought about them, and consequently to feel less inadequate than they otherwise would when faced with moral problems. This last point is added since many practising nurses (at least many of those I meet) say they feel inadequate when faced with moral problems during the course of their work. The source of this, it turns out, is often the belief that there are experts in moral philosophy around who know and can prove just what the right course of action to take in a given situation is.

Studying ethics helps to dispel this illusion and indicate to nurses that they have at least as much to offer as other groups of people in moral decision-making. In fact, the terminology of moral philosophy provides nurses with a technical vocabulary within which to couch their explanations of their own moral decisions – as might reasonably be expected of accountable professionals. It should be added that this vocabulary is one which is recognised by medical staff, health service managers, and health economists. Hence, employing the vocabulary can help nurses to voice their concerns about relevant moral matters in an effective way.

There is a useful passage from Seedhouse (1988, p. 64) which we might briefly consider here:

> The realistic aim of ethical inquiry is to clarify the issues, to show those who have to make decisions the full range of possibilities open to them, and to explain different perspectives and ways of reasoning.

Seedhouse indicates here that ethics, when applied to the health care context, has very modest aims; it cannot provide uniquely and indisputably correct solutions to moral problems.

Having now, hopefully, persuaded the reader that nurses should study ethics, a strategy for identifying moral issues will now be considered.

How can moral issues be identified?

Some moral issues seem easy to identify: for example, those concerning the rightness or wrongness of abortion, of mistreatment of persons with severe learning disabilities, and of injustices in the distribution of health care resources. But moral issues pervade nursing practice. Consider actions such as moving a person from one chair to another without speaking to the client; removing the coat from a conscious, confused client without their permission; preventing a confused, elderly client from leaving a day hospital; coercing a person with learning difficulties into having a bath, or a wash; and so on. These kinds of examples are much less likely to be cited by nursing staff as examples of moral problems encountered in practice. Yet, as will be seen below, situations such as those just described do have a moral aspect and do raise moral questions. To further sensitivity to moral issues it may be useful to describe the following strategy.

The motivation for devising this strategy stems from speaking to many student nurses who claim never to have encountered a moral issue during their clinical placements. Undoubtedly, one has to learn to recognise such issues and in this section an attempt is made to try to outline one way of overcoming the difficulties which some people have in this area. The strategy has to be consciously applied and this can require a certain determination on the part of the person concerned to put the strategy into practice. Nonetheless, many nursing students (pre and post-registration) claim to find the strategy helpful and so it is set out below in the hope that others may find it so.

It was noted earlier that ethics is concerned with certain kinds of situations and the language employed to describe these. But it seems that not all situations have an ethical aspect. The fact that Buckinghamshire is south of Manchester seems to raise no ethical concerns. We come closer to the heart of the matter when we observe that ethics is concerned with situations which involve actions. Suppose a person, Smith, pushes another person, Jones, off the edge of a cliff with the consequence that Jones is badly injured. This seems clearly to be an action about which we might make a moral judgement – for example, to the effect that Smith was wrong (or right) to push Jones off the cliff. In this example, Smith undertakes an action which results in harm to another person. Consider, now, another description of an action: Sue opens a door and closes it again for no reason and with no intention of harming anyone; the action has no effect on any person. More strictly, it needs to be supposed that the action affects no sentient individual, human or otherwise.

It is plausible to hold that the first situation has an ethical aspect whilst the second one does not. Although both examples involve actions, the action undertaken by Smith results in harm to another person – Jones. But Sue's action has no effects, harmful or beneficial, on any other person.

Consideration of these two examples suggests that the situations which are most central to the concerns of ethics include those which involve actions which result in harms or benefits to others. Jones's action qualifies as an action with an ethical aspect on this criterion, and Sue's action fails to qualify. This enables us to improve on the definition of ethics offered at the beginning of this chapter. Ethics may now be said to include enquiry into certain situations and into the language employed to describe such situations; the kinds of situations referred to are those which have led or may lead to harms or benefits to sentient individuals.

Typically, certain terms are employed, or can be employed to describe situations with an ethical aspect. Such terms include the following:

- right
- wrong
- good
- bad
- duty
- obligation
- should
- ought
- harm

and so on. For the sake of brevity, let us refer to this list henceforth as *The List*. When one hears sentences with these terms occurring in them being used, it is likely that some kind of ethical claim is being made. For example:

- That was a good (or bad) thing to do;
- You ought to act in the best interests of your patients;
- You should have intervened when you saw a man in the street being assaulted;
- It is the duty of health care professionals to prolong life where possible;
- Nurses have an obligation to protect patients;
- Patients have a right to be told the truth about their condition;
- It is not right that some people are homeless;

and so on. These sentences each include one of the terms identified in *The List*. (See Hanfling [1972] on this issue; and Hare [1952].)

Of course, some of the terms may be used in contexts which we would judge have nothing to do with ethics. For example, someone may say to a lost motorist, 'You should have turned right at the lights'. Here, the terms 'should' and 'right' occur in a context which seems not to have anything to do with ethics.

However, it is plausible to hold that, in general, when the terms in the list offered above are employed, it is often the case that some kind of ethical judgement is being made. The terms in *The List* constitute indicators that an ethical claim is being made, they are not a cast-iron guarantee of the expression of such a claim. So, one way to identify ethical situations in the health care setting is to listen out for the words in *The List*; when they are used, or when one finds oneself using them, it is likely that some kind of ethical judgement is being made.

Clearly there are many situations which arise and about which no comments are made. For example, in a hospital ward – call it ward W – in a mental health setting, it may be that clients are expected to queue up for their meals whilst these are served out by nursing staff. This routine may take place three times each day without anyone, nurse or client, passing a comment upon the nature of the routine. From the fact that nobody offers a description of this routine, it does not follow that the situation lacks an ethical aspect. What this indicates is that in applying the strategy one has not simply to listen to actual descriptions of situations offered by people (colleagues, clients or relatives of clients), one must also ask the following question: Could someone describe this situation (that being witnessed, or reflected upon) in a way which involves a sentence containing one of the terms given in *The List*?

Suppose Ann is a student nurse and has been on placement at ward W for three weeks. Nobody has passed comment upon the mealtime routine just described. Suppose further that Ann decides to apply the strategy outlined above. She asks herself the question: Could someone describe this situation (clients queuing for meals which are doled out by nursing staff) in sentences which include any of the terms on *The List*? It seems plain that another person, Beth, might say 'It's not right that clients should have to queue for their meals like that', or similarly 'It's wrong that clients are expected to queue for their meals in that way', or, again similarly, 'Clients should not be expected to queue in that way'. The possibility of Beth legitimately making observations such as these indicates that the situation has a moral aspect. The student nurse who is applying the strategy – Ann – should then consider why Beth's observations might be made; that is, are her comments justified?

An important point to note here is that whether or not the practice of expecting clients to queue for meals is justified, the fact that judgements such as those made by Beth may be made about the mealtime routine on ward W indicates that the situation does have an ethical aspect. The question of whether the routine is justified from the ethical perspective is not one which we are concerned with here. Our present task is to develop and enhance the ability of nurses to identify situations with a moral aspect. The first stage in that process involves the application of the strategy just described.

To summarise: First, one needs to listen out for the terms which feature in *The List*. If these are being employed to describe a situation (for example, the mealtime routine on ward W), it is likely some kind of ethical claim is being made and that the situation under discussion has an ethical aspect. But this first step in the strategy needs to be supplemented with a second step. The person applying the strategy needs to reflect upon the situation and ask: Could someone describe this situation in sentences which include any of the terms on *The List*? Of course, it is not plausible to apply the strategy during an emergency situation, but it is possible to apply it during quieter moments in one's spell of duty, during ward-based teaching sessions, and in any period when one is reflecting upon one's work.

This chapter may be drawn to a close by making a quite general point. It was noted earlier that actions which result in harms or benefits to others form a major part of the subject matter of ethics. Since the point of health care is to promote the well-being of patients and clients – to undertake actions which result in benefits to others – it is plausible to hold that every nursing action has an ethical aspect. This point underlies Seedhouse's slogan 'Work for health is a moral endeavour' (1988, p. 17). Since, presumably, all nursing actions – filling in records, interacting with clients and so on – are ultimately undertaken for the benefit of clients, it is evident that Seedhouse's slogan is apposite. It is true that some actions undertaken by nurses may involve causing harm to clients. Perhaps giving people medication against their will is an example, as is giving medication by injection. But these harm-causing actions are only justifiably undertaken in the belief that they will result in benefits to the client; specifically, that the benefits to the client – say, of medication – outweigh the harms which might befall the client – say, due to side effects of the medication.

2 *A principle-based approach to nursing ethics*

In the previous chapter, the nature of ethics was considered briefly and a strategy offered for the identification of moral problems which arise from nursing practice. In the present chapter, an approach to such problems is set out and discussed. In formulating the approach we will need to consider a general outline of a framework for moral reasoning, to consider two influential moral theories, and to understand the relations between the various levels of the framework. In the final sections of this chapter it will be argued that level three of the framework captures the most important level of moral thinking for our purposes, and certain strengths of a principle-based approach will be outlined.

The framework and its levels

Melia (1989, pp. 6–7) describes the following approach to moral thinking;

> First there are the particular judgements that nurses make for individual cases ... At another level there are rules which state what ought and ought not to be done ... These rules are justified by more general ... principles ... Finally, at the highest level of abstraction, there are ethical theories ...

The approach summarised here by Melia is that set out in Beauchamp and Childress (1989), but her brief statement of it is particularly helpful. It will be useful, now, to consider it more thoroughly, to attempt to indicate its use in what follows.

A first point of interest is the reference to levels of moral thinking. At what might be called level one there are 'particular judgements'; at level two there are 'rules'; at level three there are 'principles'; and at level four there are 'ethical theories'

(Melia, 1989). Each of these levels will be considered in turn, beginning with level-one judgements.

Level-one judgements

These are judgements which concern a particular situation; they are made by those involved in the situation, those who witness the situation or those who simply read or come to hear about it. One example of a moral judgement may consist of a decision by a nurse to withhold information from a client. Perhaps the client asks the nurse for information concerning the side effects of medication presently being prescribed. The nurse might judge that it is best or right to withhold this information on the grounds that if the client learns the truth he might refuse to take the medication with the probable consequence (in the nurse's view) that the client's condition will worsen.

Another example of a particular moral judgement is, say, a nurse's judgement that the client's request for information concerning the side effects of his medication should be responded to in a different way. The considerations of the previous chapter support the conclusion that all actions undertaken by nursing staff can be said to have a moral aspect. This indicates that all decisions or judgements made by nurses also have a moral aspect, since such decisions are decisions to act in one way as opposed to another. In the example just given, the nurse is required to make a particular moral judgement: should the client be given the information requested or not? A situation such as this demands that the nurse makes a moral judgement.

It might be suggested that the nurse could simply avoid making a judgement, perhaps by informing the client that he or she (the nurse) does not have the information, or is not able to give the information. But even strategies such as these also have a moral component since, presumably, the nurse thinks that either the client or the nurse will be harmed if the information is given (perhaps the nurse has been 'instructed' by medical staff not to give the information to the client). The point is that even a judgement not to make a decision – an evasion, so to speak – is also a decision to act in a way which has a moral aspect. This is due to the fact that considerations involving possible harms and benefits, either to the client or the nurse concerned, enter into the basis for the decision.

The example just discussed is intended to explicate the notion of a moral judgement. Recall that, in the approach to moral thinking described in the quote from Melia (1989) given above, such judgements occur at a level which can be described as level-one. Consider, now, another level.

Level-two rules

At the next level, level two, it is proposed, '[That] there are rules which state what ought and ought not to be done . . . ' (Melia, 1989). The example of such a rule which Melia provides is, '[It] is wrong to lie'. There are two important points which need to be made here.

The first is that a particular moral judgement is an instance of a moral rule. The relationship between rules and their instances can be explained as follows. Suppose one is driving a car and stops at a red light. This particular act of stopping at a red light is an instance of the driver obeying the rule 'Stop at red lights'. So, for example, not lying to a client, or telling the truth to a client, can plausibly be regarded as instancing the general rules 'It is wrong to lie', or, 'One ought to be truthful'.

The second important point here is that level-two rules provide justification for level-one judgements (cf. Beauchamp and Childress, 1989, p. 7). Hence, if asked to justify an act of telling a client the truth (as in our earlier example), a nurse may say that one ought to tell the truth, or it is wrong to lie to others. The nurse appeals to level-two rules as justifications for the act – the act of telling a client the truth.

Are there examples of other rules? Beauchamp and Childress refer specifically to four. These are the rules of veracity, privacy, confidentiality and fidelity (1989, ch. 7).

The veracity rule

By a rule of veracity, Beauchamp and Childress mean a rule to the effect that one is under '[An] obligation to tell the truth and not to lie or deceive others' (1989, p. 307). Hence, in the health care context, the rule of veracity requires that one should be truthful in one's interactions with clients (and colleagues), and one should not deceive them. When applied to our earlier example, the rule of veracity generates an obligation to tell the client the truth and to supply him with the information he has requested.

The privacy rule

Beauchamp and Childress define privacy as '[A] state or condition of limited access to a person' (1989, p. 319). Hence, a rule of privacy generates an obligation to respect what might be described as the 'personal space' of an individual. This can be understood in at least two ways. First, quite literally, in terms of an obligation not to encroach upon a person – perhaps by entering the person's home without invitation. Application of the privacy rule seems especially relevant to the context of working with clients who have learning disabilities. For example, as some new community home is opened – say, one which contains some special facility – a procession of visitors are often shown round the new home. Such visitors may include local dignitaries or other workers in the field of learning disabilities. It is plausible that such visits constitute violations of the privacy rule in this first sense. (Think how most people would respond to having strangers shown around their homes.) And second, respecting the privacy of the person can take the form of restricting access to information about the person. So, for example, a nurse who gives out information concerning a client without the client's permission can plausibly be regarded as breaching the privacy of that client. This second aspect of the privacy rule is, of course, closely related to the confidentiality rule.

The confidentiality rule

This is defined by Beauchamp and Childress as follows:

> An infringement of X's confidentiality occurs only if the person to whom X disclosed the information in confidence fails to protect that information or deliberately discloses it to someone without X's consent. (1989, p. 329)

Hence, the distinction between violating the privacy rule (in the second sense of privacy denoted earlier) and violating the confidentiality rule can be illustrated in the following two examples.

1. A client, Carol, requests that the information that she has epilepsy is not passed on to her employers should they ever enquire. A nurse passes this information on to Carol's employers when they request it. This example constitutes a breach of the confidentiality rule since Carol specifically requested that this information should not be given to her employers. (The question of whether this is a justified breach of confidentiality can, of course, still be raised.)
2. Carol is a client on ward W, as before; Carol has epilepsy and has been admitted to hospital due to the fact that she has recently experienced a large number of major seizures. Carol has not made any specific request that information concerning her condition should not be passed on to other parties (for example, her employers). Carol's employers ring the ward enquiring how she is and how long she is likely to be off work. During this enquiry, her employers ask what the nature of Carol's illness is. The nurse dealing with the enquiry informs Carol's employers that it is Carol's epilepsy which is the reason for her admission to hospital. The nurse who passes such information on breaches the privacy rule.

We shall return to discuss the confidentiality rule later, but now move on to consider the fourth and final level-two moral rule identified by Beauchamp and Childress.

The fidelity rule
This is understood as a rule relating to promise-keeping. Hence, the fidelity rule generates an obligation to keep promises made to clients.

In the nursing context, the rule can be taken to apply in at least two senses. The most obvious arises when nurses make explicit promises to clients. A nurse might promise that she will return to see a client the following day – perhaps the client is in need of this reassurance. Or, a nurse might promise a client detained under the mental health act that she will accompany them to the local shops later in the day if the client is not considered well enough to go unescorted. It is evident that there are numerous scenarios in which it is possible that a nurse might make an explicit promise to a client to undertake some task or other. Clearly, there is an obligation in such circumstances to keep one's promises.

A second sense of the application of the fidelity rule concerns implicit promises. One apparent example of situations in which there are implicit promises on the part of nurses to clients arises in contexts in which clients give information about themselves to nurses. Clients give information such as their age, next of kin and so forth, on the tacit understanding that the nurse concerned will convey the information only to parties who have a legitimate interest – namely, other health care professionals (medical staff, other nurses and so on). Further, it is plausible to assert that clients assume that nursing staff implicitly promise to undertake their duties with the required degree of skill and care, to provide them with relevant information and not to be wilfully negligent.

These, then, are the four level-two moral rules identified by Beauchamp and Childress. It should be clear that the example of a moral rule offered by Melia ('It is wrong to lie' – 1989, p. 6) can be subsumed within the veracity rule; so too can rules such as, 'One ought, in general, to tell the truth'. We will return shortly to comment on the relationship between level-two moral rules and clauses in the UKCC Code of Conduct (UKCC, 1992). Before this, it is necessary to look, briefly, at four level-three principles (these are to be set out more fully in Chapter 3), and at two level-four moral theories.

Level-three principles

In Beauchamp and Childress's framework, four moral principles are referred to. These are the principle of respect for *autonomy*, the principle of *beneficence*, the principle of *nonmaleficence*, and the principle of *justice*. Principles are claimed to be more general than moral rules. For example, the principle of nonmaleficence points to obligations not to harm. This is clearly more general than specific moral rules such as: do not burn others; do not hit them, and so on. So the sense in which principles are more general than rules seems fairly easy to grasp.

Summarily stated, the principle of respect for *autonomy* generates an obligation to respect the choices which others make concerning their own lives. Hence, if a cognitively competent client chooses, on the basis of relevant information, not to take medication prescribed, then the principle of respect for autonomy generates an obligation on the part of others to respect that choice.

The principle of *beneficence* generates an obligation to act in ways which promote the well-being of others. It is clear that construed in this way, this principle is of central relevance to the nursing context and, more generally, to all health care workers. As we saw in Chapter 1, the point of nursing actions is to promote the well-being of clients and, hence, to act in accord with the principle of beneficence.

The principle of *nonmaleficence* generates obligations not to harm others. This differs from beneficence in the sense that it imposes fewer obligations on others. For example, suppose one is walking down a city street and one sees a person who is obviously thin, unhealthy and hungry. The principle of beneficence generates obligations to help this person, to act in ways which will benefit him. But nonmaleficence is less morally demanding, so to speak: it only generates obligations not to harm the person.

The distinction between the principles of beneficence and nonmaleficence has quite serious implications for health care professionals. Presumably, a fundamental aim of health care is, as suggested above, to promote the well-being of clients. Hence, as we noted, the actions of nursing staff can be said to be grounded in beneficence. So it is reasonable to conclude that regimes of care should actually benefit clients, rather than simply not cause harm. Thus, regimes of care which merely prevent harm befalling their clients fall short of what is required by the principle of beneficence.

The fourth and final level-four principle to be defined briefly here is the principle of *justice*. Crudely, this principle generates obligations to treat others fairly. On one construal, this principle asserts that equals be treated equally (cf. Beauchamp and Childress, 1989, p. 257). So, in the nursing context, suppose in one set of circumstances a nurse tells the truth to a client, Colin, at his request, concerning the nature of his condition. Later, a client, Charles, whose circumstances are the same as Colin's makes a similar request. This time the nurse fobs the client off and does not give Charles the information he requests – it is to be assumed that the nurse has time to speak to Charles. Since the situations of Colin and Charles in our example are the same, Charles may claim that he has not been treated fairly and that the principle of justice has been transgressed.

This brings this preliminary introduction to the four level-three moral principles to a close. Moving on, two level-four moral theories will now be discussed – specifically, Utilitarianism and a Kantian duty-based or deontological theory.

Level-four moral theories: (i) Utilitarianism

It is possible to identify two influential moral theories: a first which focuses upon the consequences of actions and which, hence, can be described as consequence-based; and a second which focuses on moral duty and which can be described as duty-based. The first of these theories is termed Utilitarianism (two of its most famous proponents were J. Bentham [1748–1832] and J. S. Mill [1808–73]).

With regard to the issue of truth-telling, a nurse who is a Utilitarian would base a decision concerning which course of action to take on a consideration of the consequences of those actions. So, in the event of a choice between truth-telling and not truth-telling, a Utilitarian would consider the consequences of the act. An act which is morally right is the act which brings about the desired consequence.

According to the Utilitarian approach to ethics, in the event of there being a choice between two or more possible courses of action (for example, truth-telling or not), the morally correct act is that which results in the greatest 'good' for the greatest number. By 'good', here, is meant some kind of benefit – perhaps pleasure, or happiness. So, if one act, A, will result in more benefits than another act, B, then A is morally preferable to B.

In cases where all conceivable courses of action are likely to result in some degree of suffering (say, the case of a terminally ill person who is in constant pain; or a person with mental health problems who is tormented by hallucinations), Utilitarianism demands that the morally correct act is that which results in the least amount of harms – the least amount of pain and suffering.

Thus, according to Utilitarians, acts are morally right to the extent that they either maximise benefits (say, happiness) or minimise harms. This is captured in the so-called principle of utility:

> [Actions] are right in proportion as they tend to promote happiness, wrong as they tend to produce the reverse of happiness. By happiness is intended pleasure, and the absence of pain; by unhappiness, pain and the privation of pleasure. (Mill, 1861, p. 257)

Before continuing further, pause to consider some possible points in favour of Utilitarianism. First, the approach seeks to establish a quantifiable basis for moral decision-making by employing a kind of calculation. Thus, moral decision-making would not be a matter of arbitrary opinion, but would be based on calculation. In support of this feature, Beauchamp and Childress offer the following example. By the early 1980s, success rates for heart transplants were relatively high (at Stanford University, 65 per cent of selected patients survived at least one year and had a 'better than 50 per cent' chance of surviving five years). Some claimed that the heart transplant programme should be expanded in the light of these success rates – though there were still worries voiced concerning tissue rejection and other issues. On 1 February 1980, the 12 lay trustees of Massachusetts General Hospital voted not to allow heart transplants at that hospital. They said they had a 'clear responsibility to evaluate new procedures in terms of the greatest good for the greatest number'. The worry of the trustees was that since heart transplants are so expensive (and that the claimed success rates were still viewed with some scepticism), the cost of performing them would mean that less money would be available for other aspects of health care provision. Many people, presumably, benefited from these other services. So, in deciding not to permit heart transplants, the trustees can be seen to have placed the greatest benefit of the greatest number above a great benefit for a smaller number – this being an example of Utilitarian reasoning in a health care setting (example taken from Beauchamp and Childress, 1989, pp. 446–9). Second, the claim that acts are morally right if they maximise happiness or minimise suffering seems, at least at first sight, to be a plausible one. Most of us would agree that happiness is a good thing which should be promoted, and that suffering is an undesirable phenomenon which should be diminished.

Third, a further consideration in support of Utilitarianism is this: in duty-based ethical theory, one of the most quoted duties is that of being truthful. However, there seem to be occasions where one might think it unwise to be truthful. Consider a case in which a person, A, intends to injure another person, B; you know where B is; you also know that if you reveal B's whereabouts, then B will take a severe beating. It seems wrong in such a case to tell the truth to A, especially if you know that in an hour or so A will have calmed down and will not want to assault B. An apparent advantage of Utilitarianism is that some flexibility appears to be present in such cases. If it is the case that not telling the truth results in more happiness, then we would be justified in not telling the truth. So, in our example, it would be acceptable to lie and so save B from a beating.

These three sets of considerations indicate that Utilitarianism has at least an initial plausibility. It is common to distinguish two forms of Utilitarianism: Act Utilitarianism and Rule Utilitarianism.

Act Utilitarianism

Act Utilitarians consider only the consequences of one act at a time. So, when they face a moral dilemma, they will simply calculate which of the possible acts will maximise benefits or minimise harms. One of the criticisms of this theory is the following (adapted from Smart and Williams, 1973, p. 69). In the USA in the 19th and 20th centuries a number of so-called race riots took place as a result of racial tension. Suppose that in one of the areas where there is a great deal of racial tension a crime is committed which heightens the tension. Perhaps a white person is killed by a black person. The white community hears about this and demands that someone is arrested and given the death penalty. The local police decide simply to arrest and frame a person selected entirely at random. By doing this, they prevent a riot taking place in which hundreds of people might have been killed. Such a course of action seems to be in complete accord with Act Utilitarianism since it placates the crowd, and the riot does not take place: the death of one person prevents the death of hundreds.

However, the fact that the performance of such an apparently unjust act seems justifiable in Act Utilitarianism may be taken to constitute a powerful criticism of it – it seems morally abhorrent to punish an innocent person. So another form of Utilitarianism – Rule Utilitarianism – has been proposed to overcome the kind of objection presented by the race-riot case.

Rule Utilitarianism

In response to the race-riot example, it may have occurred to the reader that although arresting the innocent person is a utility in the short term, in the longer term it would be a disutility (it would not lead to more benefits than harms). For example, it could be pointed out that respect for the law would decline if it was the case that innocent persons could be charged for crimes they have not committed. On the assumption that respect for the law is a desirable goal, one may conclude that there is a long-term general utility in upholding the moral rule that innocent persons should not be punished for crimes they have not committed. So, certain moral rules should be respected due to the fact that their adoption leads to more good consequences than bad.

What seems to be violated in the race-riot example is the view that it is morally wrong to punish innocent people. As a result, Rule Utilitarians would attempt to introduce adherence to such rules while remaining faithful to the basic Utilitarian principle of maximising happiness and minimising harm. Rule Utilitarianism would recognise that arresting an innocent person may prevent the riot, but since that would involve transgressing the moral rule that innocent persons should not be punished, the Rule Utilitarian can avoid the objection. Other examples of rules which a Rule Utilitarian might propose are: (i) Do not lie;

(ii) Do not kill; (iii) Do not steal; and so on. They would claim that adherence to these rules leads to more benefits than harms.

So, for the Rule Utilitarian, rules which lead to the maximisation of pleasure should be adhered to. Consider truth-telling again: from the Rule Utilitarian perspective it may be proposed that health care professionals should be truthful with their clients. The reason, it may be said, is that clients are more likely to trust health care professionals if they are sure that they are honest and truthful. In this case, they will be more likely to impart relevant information and hold such professionals in high regard. It can be supposed that these consequences of being truthful are beneficial (lead to more good consequences than bad consequences), since health care professionals often require information in order to treat clients successfully; and if they are held in high regard, their views are likely to be respected. So, even if on a particular occasion being truthful with a client leads to more harmful than beneficial consequences, the net benefits of being truthful might be claimed to outweigh the net harms.

It is therefore conceivable that a Rule Utilitarian may tell the truth to a client even if, on that occasion, doing so leads to more harms than benefits. They would do so on the grounds that adherence to a moral rule which requires that one is truthful with others, generally leads to more benefits than harms.

Having looked at the general character of Utilitarianism, and also at the distinction between Act and Rule Utilitarianism, some of the common criticisms of this position will now be considered.

Criticism of Utilitarianism

Although the Utilitarian claims to provide a secure basis for moral decision-making, it is not clear that that is what is provided in practice. It is of course notoriously difficult to determine the consequences of particular acts or of the adoption of general rules. For example, suppose an Act Utilitarian refrains from telling the truth to a client on the grounds that so doing would be a disutility. Say, for example, that one of the client's children has died unknown to the client, and the utilitarian doctor, believing that the client has only a few days to live, does not want to burden the client with this news even when he is asked by the client if his children are well. If the client were to get better, he might become extremely distressed about the fact that he was lied to; and this may sour the future relationship between health care professionals and that client.

Second, Williams (1972) argues that Utilitarianism is morally debasing. Since its sole aim is the maximising of pleasure (or minimising of pain), in principle, any act could be said to be morally correct. The point being, here, that in some other moral theories certain types of acts are claimed to be absolutely wrong, with a clear restriction on what is permissible. In Utilitarianism, however, the overriding consideration is maximising utility, so that it is possible that an act which might be considered morally abhorrent would be morally permissible in Utilitarianism – even torturing babies or young children. Nothing is ruled out, it seems.

Third, in the health care setting, it could be argued that adoption of Utilitarian ethics encourages acceptance of states of affairs which perhaps should be questioned. For example, a hospital manager might consider how best to use his small numbers of nursing staff and apply Utilitarian considerations to the problem. However, it could be suggested that the question that should be addressed is that of why there are such limited resources – that is, as opposed to simply deciding what is the best way to allocate existing resources in accord with a Utilitarian view.

Fourth, Williams points out that from the Utilitarian perspective certain acts seem obviously right. For example, suppose one could save the lives of ten people but only by killing one person. Even if that is indeed morally right, Williams wonders whether it is *obviously* right (Williams, cited in Smart and Williams, 1973, p. 98). So, in spite of initial attractions, it appears that there are certain serious worries which accompany wholesale endorsement of Utilitarianism.

Level-four moral theories: (ii) a deontological theory

Deontological theories of ethics take duty to be the basis of morality. It is, though, important to distinguish professional duty from moral duty. Professional duties are stated in the UKCC Code of Conduct (UKCC, 1992), but moral duties are not. However, as will be seen, moral duties can plausibly be claimed to underlie professional duties.

Perhaps the most well-known form of deontological moral theory is that proposed by Immanual Kant (1724–1804). His view is stated in his *Groundwork of the Metaphysic of Morals*, which can be found in Paton (1948). (For references to other versions of deontological theories see Beauchamp and Childress, 1989, p. 37; and Singer, 1991.) Kant is without doubt one of the most important of philosophers but his work is notoriously difficult and there are various interpretations of it. Despite this, his *Groundwork* is well worth reading; it is quite a short book and one of the classics of moral philosophy.

From our point of view, Kant's theory has relevance due to its emphasis on duty where this is considered apart from consequences. Many moral agents hold that certain courses of action are definitely morally wrong, regardless of their consequences, and that it is a weakness of Utilitarianism that no type of action is definitely ruled out; as we saw, this is because in Utilitarianism the overriding considerations centre on maximisation of utility. Further, Kant's theory allocates a central role to the notion of *autonomy*; and the principle of respect for autonomy is regarded by many commentators as one of the most important principles in ethics as it applies to the health care setting (see, for example, Chapter 3 following; Downie and Calman, 1987; Beauchamp and Childress, 1989; Seedhouse, 1988; and Harris, 1985).

Kant's moral theory begins from an acceptance of the view that there is a moral theory currently in place; that is, there is a moral system which people generally employ – call this the 'commonsense' theory, or 'ordinary moral thought'. His view seems to be that any moral theory should reflect the main components of the commonsense theory. So, for Kant, there is an existing moral system in place which people apply, in rough and ready fashion, in their ordinary dealings with each other. What he seeks to do is to propose a moral theory which rests upon the fundamental components of this ongoing, commonsense theory. As Kant puts it:

The sole aim of the present Groundwork is to seek out and establish *the supreme principle of morality* . . . The method I have adopted
. . . [proceeds] analytically from common knowledge to the foundation of its supreme principle and then back again synthetically
from an examination of this principle and its origins to the
common knowledge in which we find its application. (Paton, 1948,
pp. 57–8; also Raphael, 1981, p. 58)

Kant notes that there is a particular distinction which is present
in ordinary moral thought and which is regarded as important
within such thought. He draws attention to a distinction between acts which are done out of respect for duty on the one
hand, and acts done either from what he calls inclination or
acts done from prudential considerations (acting out of self-
interest) on the other. (See, for example, Kant's discussion of
the 'shopkeeper': p. 63.) Kant's view can be put thus:

A human action is morally good, not because it is done from
immediate inclination – still less because it is done from self-interest – but because it is done for the sake of duty. (Paton, 1948, p. 19,
summarising Kant's view)

So, in the following three cases, there is alleged to be a moral
difference between the actors:

1. A person, A, who acts out of respect for duty, performs an
   act of type X because he takes it to be the case that he has a
   duty to do X – regardless of the consequences (as in the case
   of truth-telling, for example). In the nursing context, we
   may suppose that A is a student nurse Alan, who notices
   that a severely physically disabled client has been incontinent and acts to make the client comfortable by helping him
   to change into dry clothing. Alan does this act out of recognition of a moral duty to help people unable to help themselves where possible.
2. A person, B, who performs an act of type X (as before,
   telling the truth, or being honest) merely out of conveni-
   ence and not out of any particular recognition of a duty to
   do X (to be truthful). Such a person is said by Kant to be
   acting out of inclination (p. 63). He may do X just as person,
   A, above, but although his action is in accord with duty, it

is not done out of respect for duty. For example, suppose that Alan had made the client referred to in case (1) comfortable simply to fill in some time and not from of an intention to act morally: Alan's action would be in accord with moral duty, but would not be undertaken out of respect for moral duty.

3. A person, C, who performs an act of type X for purely prudential reasons – purely from self-interest. Kant gives the example of a shopkeeper who is honest because he or she fears that there may be adverse consequences of not being honest – the acquiring of a bad reputation and loss of business, for example (p. 63). Such a person is honest only because of calculating the consequences of not being honest, and concluding that it is not in their best interests to be dishonest. Again, of such a person, it can be claimed that they act in accord with duty but not out of respect for duty. Another example would be a student nurse who makes comfortable the client referred to in cases (1) and (2) simply to impress the charge nurse; this would qualify as acting out of self-interest rather than from moral duty.

Kant suggests, plausibly, that a moral difference can be identified between the actor in 1 and the actor in 2 and 3. What is central to the distinction is the intentions of the actors: A intends to act in accord with duty but this is not the case with B and C. Kant especially seeks to emphasise the difference between A and C. C's decision to act honestly is the consequence of reasoning *hypothetically*. That is, he reasons thus: 'if I do X the consequences will be Y; if I do not do X, the consequences will be Z. Since I desire Y, I'll do X'. In the case of A, however, Kant points out that he does not go through such a reasoning process; A simply reasons thus: 'it is my duty to do X, therefore I ought to do X'. (See, for example, Kant, p. 78, on the difference between reasoning hypothetically and reasoning categorically.)

As mentioned earlier, a central component in Kant's theory is the concept of *autonomy* (see, for example, p. 93), and it is important to say a few words about this before continuing. As noted, Kant takes as fundamental the distinction between acting out of respect for duty, and acting in accord with duty. To be capable of acting out of respect for duty it is necessary that the person is free to decide to act in such a way. So, Kant's view requires that what he calls 'the will' (the mind) is actually free to make moral decisions.

This should be easy for us to accept: ordinary moral thought distinguishes an act done voluntarily from one done as a result of coercion. For example, suppose two people donate half of their savings to a worthwhile charity. It is later discovered that one did this of his own free will whilst the other did it because he was under some kind of threat – suppose he was blackmailed into donating the sum to charity. Commonsense moral thinking would distinguish between the two acts: the view being that the voluntary donation is the more worthy act from the moral perspective. This example indicates the central position which the notion of autonomy has in moral thought. In fact, autonomy seems to be a necessary condition of the possibility of morality. This is certainly something which Kant wants to claim; and, as noted, many commentators on health care ethics place heavy emphasis on the notion of autonomy (Downie and Calman, 1987; Harris, 1985).

A further point which needs to be mentioned here is that in drawing the distinction between hypothetical and categorical reasoning, the subject who reasons hypothetically takes into consideration facts which for Kant are not relevant to the question of the rightness or otherwise of the particular act. Instead of simply thinking about what it is his duty to do the subject who reasons hypothetically considers the consequences of his act. For Kant, thinking in such a way constitutes a threat to the person's autonomy; when subjects 'look beyond' the question of what is right or wrong and begin to consider the consequences of their acts they are not thinking morally – he says they are looking for 'inducements' (p. 67) to act morally; and moral actions are not undertaken out of consideration of 'inducements'. Hence, the difference between Kant's duty-based approach to ethics, and the Utilitarian approach can be seen to be extremely profound.

The categorical imperative

Kant takes it to be the case that acting morally is essentially bound up with acting out of respect for duty. In fact, he is claiming that it is a necessary condition of moral actions that they are carried out due to recognition of duty. Given this claim, then, concerning the necessity of the notion of duty to moral reasoning, the question arises of which particular duties we ought to decide, as individual autonomous persons, to respect. (Bear in mind that for Kant these have to be worked out for oneself.)

Kant claims that we can determine what our duty is by applying the categorical imperative (it is claimed to be categorical because it admits of no exceptions; and it is claimed to be imperative because it is necessary – according to Kant – to act out of respect for it):

> I ought never to act except in such a way that I can also will that my maxim should become a universal law. (Kant, p. 67)

Put less formally: do unto others as you would have them do unto you. Roughly, the claim is that one should only perform an act of type X (not telling the truth; not keeping a promise; telling the truth; keeping a promise) if one is prepared to allow that every other person in similar circumstances should necessarily perform the same type of act. So, if a person tells a lie he should be prepared to allow it to be the case that lying should become a universal law, that everyone must lie. Kant takes it to be self-evident that the latter state of affairs is sufficiently disagreeable that everyone would see it as unacceptable (cf. Kant's *Groundwork*, p. 85).

Note that Kant's imperative does seem to be a central feature of commonsense morality. Often we try to appeal to people's moral sense by saying, 'What would the world be like if everyone acted like that?' For example, one might try to get a child to start to think in this way: if he were to steal another child's toy we might say, 'What if everyone behaved like you?' – the implication being that no one would actually have any toys of their own.

Kant provides the following illustration of the categorical imperative in action:

> A man feels sick of life as the result of a series of misfortunes that has mounted to the point of despair,but he is still so far in posses-

sion of his reason as to ask himself whether taking his own life may not be contrary to his duty to himself. He now applies the test 'Can the maxim of my action really become a universal law of nature?' His maxim is 'From self-love I make it my principle to shorten my life if its continuance threatens more evil than it promises pleasure'. The only further question to ask is whether this principle of self-love can become a universal law of nature. It is then seen at once that a system of nature by whose law the very same feeling whose function is to stimulate the furtherance of life should actually destroy life would contradict itself and consequently could not subsist as a system of nature. Hence this maxim cannot possibly hold as a universal law of nature and is therefore entirely opposed to the supreme principle of all duty [that is, the categorical imperative]. (Kant, p. 85)

It can be seen from the above passage that an important feature of the categorical imperative is its relationship to the notion of autonomy. To apply it, it is necessary to consider the perspectives of other people. It is necessary to put oneself in the position of other autonomous beings. In the above quote, the thinker appears to conclude that if he thinks it morally right to end his life if it looks like that life is going to involve much pain and suffering, then it will be a universal law that others who reach the same conclusion should then end their lives also. Crudely, for Kant, 'self-love' seems to amount to something like 'self-preservation', or 'self-regard'. Hence, suicide in Kant's view can be seen to be acting in contradiction to his maxim, which urges him both to prolong his life and to shorten it.

A further, famous formulation of the categorical imperative is this:

Act in such a way that you always treat humanity, whether in thine own person or in that of any other, never simply as a means, but always at the same time as an end. (p. 91)

This states that other humans are autonomous, rational moral agents and should be respected as such. So, according to this statement, institutions such as slavery are morally wrong because they involve treating humans as tools – as a means to the promotion of others' ends. Hence, it can be seen that it is not a criticism of a person's moral standards to say that he uses tools (hammers, screwdrivers and so on), but it is a criticism to say that a person uses other people.

Along roughly similar lines, it could be said that institutions such as battery farming involve treating chickens as means and not as ends; we don't take into account the well-being of the chickens but merely use them for our own ends.

Evidently, this formulation of Kant's imperative raises the distinction between categorical and hypothetical reasoning again. In reasoning categorically, a subject thinks simply, 'I ought to do X'. But in using another person to further our own ends we are reasoning hypothetically: 'I desire X; to bring about X, I need S to do Y'.

Comments on Kantian theory

Kant's emphasis on the motives and intentions of the actor seems obviously correct. Evaluation of the intentions of the actor is of relevance to evaluating the moral character of certain actions. Recall the example given earlier between the two men who make the donations to charity; we distinguish between the moral character of the actions of the two men. The further relevance of intentions is evident in law: if a person performs an act intentionally, from premeditation, he is considered more culpable than a person who commits the same act unintentionally (note the distinction between murder and manslaughter).

Also, the distinction between acting in accord with duty and acting out of respect for duty again seems to carry great plausibility. It is, furthermore, central to moral thought. Ordinary, or commonsense, moral thought clearly distinguishes between a student nurse who makes an incontinent client comfortable due to recognition of a moral obligation to do so, and a student nurse who performs the same act solely to impress the charge nurse.

In addition, the point that moral theories should respect the central components in the commonsense theory seems to be one of great importance. It seems to be the case that the commonsense theory will always be the tribunal or testing ground against which the deliverations of moral theories will be assessed. If a theorist claimed to have devised a moral theory which radically conflicted with the commonsense theory, would it be accepted? (cf. Beauchamp and Childress, 1989, p. 15).

(It should be stressed, though, that this is not to say that, for Kant, moral theory should merely reflect ordinary moral thought: see, for example, Kant, in Paton, 1948, p. 73.)

Some criticisms

Throughout the exposition of Kant's theory, reference has been made to 'the commonsense theory' or to ordinary moral thought, and it has been said that this provides a starting point for Kant. But there are at least two difficulties which follow from reliance on commonsense moral theory. First, the commonsense view of moral matters which informed Kant's thought is one which existed in 18th century Europe. Is it the case that the categorical imperative still occupies the central position in moral thinking which Kant claims for it (even if it did then)? Second, even if it is accepted that commonsense moral thought has not substantially changed in bare essentials, does it in fact conform to the demands of the categorical imperative? Take truth-telling, for example. Is it generally believed to be the case that one should always tell the truth? Or are there exceptions?

A commonly supposed counter-example to Kant's view is presented by a case in which:

> [A] maniac armed with a revolver comes looking for a relative in order to kill him. [We] would consider it highly immoral to inform the maniac of the whereabouts of the relative, merely because one ought to tell the truth. (Popkin and Stroll, 1969, p. 44)

It is not clear that this is a genuine counter-example to Kant's view, for the 'maniac' is not an autonomous moral agent. Kant's position may allow that in similar circumstances it is acceptable not to be truthful. This is because it can be allowed that a subject can think to himself, 'Can I will that my action become universal law?' and decide that it can.

A further criticism is that the theory is too rigid and therefore is inappropriate in the health care setting. Seedhouse points out that there may be situations in which it is justifiable to lie. For example, if a man has been involved in a car crash and he is badly injured, Seedhouse suggests that it may be acceptable not to tell the man the truth that his wife and children have been killed in the crash. This should be kept from him until the man is in a less critical condition (Seedhouse, 1988, pp. 100–1).

Another criticism is more theoretical. It may be claimed that the theory involves tacit appeals to consequences. For example, in the lengthy quote given earlier, Kant seems to acknowledge that the thinker should consider the consequences of everyone acting as he wants to. This seemed to be the case in the example offered of the child and the stealing of toys.

However, Kant can be defended again. The 'maxims' he refers to do include consideration of consequences (what if everyone stole private property and so on); but these maxims are not purely formal like the categorical imperative. So, at the level of principles (at the level of the categorical imperative) there is no appeal to consequences, but at the level of maxims there is. The criticism just voiced would only be decisive if it applied at the level of principles – which it does not.

A final criticism arises from the lengthy quote offered earlier concerning the person who considers taking his own life. It seems possible that a person might consider that life in general would end if everyone behaved as he did, but refuse to accept that this is self-evidently absurd. Such a person might well be prepared to universalise the maxim which Kant refers to in the passage (such a person might be described as a 'sincere nihilist').

It should be added here that just as Utilitarianism proved divisible into Act Utilitarianism and Rule Utilitarianism, so too may duty-based (deontological) moral theory (see, for example, Beauchamp and Childress, 1989, pp. 40–1). The Act Deontologist simply considers application of the categorical imperative to each particular moral problem. The Rule Deontologist, as may be anticipated, instead derives general rules from the categorical imperative. These perform the same function as what have been described here as level-two rules, or more generally, level-three principles.

The relationships between the levels of the framework

Thus far, level-one moral judgements and level-two moral rules have been considered; level-three moral principles have been briefly mentioned; and, in more depth, two major moral theories have been discussed – which, as noted, arise at level four in Beauchamp and Childress's approach. What remains now, in this chapter, is to attempt an explanation of how all these levels of theorising fit together.

Justificatory anchors

It was pointed out earlier that, in the framework, each level provides justification for the level below it. Hence, judgements are justified by rules, rules are justified by principles, and principles by level-four theories. So, the main burden of justification for any judgement appears, ultimately, to be borne by the relevant level-four theory. Let it be said that such a theory provides a justificatory anchor for judgements made through application of the framework. Suppose, first, it is considered that Utilitarianism provides such a justificatory anchor – for judgements made which employ Beauchamp and Childress's framework.

It was noted that two main versions of Utilitarianism can be identified: Act and Rule. An Act Utilitarian would clearly have no need to recruit any levels between level-one judgements and level-four theories. The Act Utilitarian would simply employ Utilitarian theory at level four, in justification of any level-one judgement. Such a theorist simply omits levels two and three.

Consider now a Rule Utilitarian. Such a theorist would attempt to justify level-one judgements by appeal to level-two rules, the justification for these being the level-four theory, Utilitarianism. Such a Rule Utilitarian omits level-three principles and simply moves from level-one judgements, to level-two rules to level four.

Alternatively, a Rule Utilitarian might consider that level-three principles provide a justification for level-two rules. Such a theorist, thus, holds that judgements are justified by rules, which in turn are justified by principles, which in turn are justified due to the fact that their application serves to maximise utility.

It can be proposed, here, that it is the latter construal of a utilitarian application of the framework which is the more plausible of the three so far described. This is due to three main reasons. First, *The Patient's Charter* (Department of Health, 1991) is expressed in terms which suggest that its foundations lie in the principles of respect for autonomy and beneficence (more on this later). Second, the same two principles (respect for autonomy and beneficence) can plausibly be shown to underpin many clauses in the UKCC Code of Conduct (again, more on this later). And third, the principles which figure in level three of Beauchamp and Childress's framework form the basis of much current work on health care ethics (see Gillon, 1994). We may therefore proceed on the presumption that a Rule Utilitarianism of the kind described in the previous paragraph is that most likely to be put forward by a proponent of a Utilitarian approach to health care ethics.

It should be clear, then, that for the Utilitarian any rules which occur at level two occur solely due to the belief that their adoption maximises utility. And, any principles which occur at level three, similarly, occur solely due to the belief that their adoption maximises utility.

So far, the question of what should be done when a conflict arises between principles has not been considered. Suppose, for example, that a client refuses potentially life-saving treatment. Here, the principle of respect for autonomy comes into conflict with the principle of beneficence (and perhaps also the principle of nonmaleficence). Respect for autonomy generates an obligation to respect the views of other persons, especially views which concern their preferences. Beneficence, on the other hand, generates obligations to promote well-being; hence, the principle of beneficence seems to generate an obligation to act in ways which will prevent the client's death.

An Act Utilitarian would try to evaluate which course of action maximises utility. This is no easy task. Perhaps it might be thought that treating the client against his wishes will serve to maximise utility. But suppose the client strongly resists such enforced treatment and dies in the struggle.

For Rule Utilitarians the situation is different. Recall that for them, right action consists in acting in accord with rules or principles the adoption of which serves to maximise utility. Therefore, the Rule Utilitarian position is one in which it would be legitimate to respect the client's wishes even if the client dies as a result of non-treatment. Such a course of action would be held to be justified if and only if, in general, respecting autonomy could be shown to result in more desirable than undesirable outcomes.

What of the duty-based approach conceived of as a justificatory anchor for Beauchamp and Childress's framework? (Recall that we are discussing moral and not professional duty.) A proponent of the duty-based approach, it would seem to me, must be committed to affording greatest weight to the principle of respect for autonomy. This is due to the centrality accorded to the concept of autonomy in the duty-based position. As seen earlier, autonomy is a necessary condition of morality in the duty-based position, and implementation of the categorical imperative requires that one consider the perspectives of other autonomous agents. Hence, the categorical imperative would form the justificatory anchor of judgements made; and in the event of a conflict between level-three principles, autonomy would always win out – providing no harms to others ensue. In the example referred to earlier, the client's decision to refuse life-saving treatment would have to be respected.

As to the distinction between Act and Rule versions of duty-based theory, Act Deontologists move straight from level-one moral judgements to the categorical imperative at level four. Rule Deontologists either formulate level-two moral rules, or, more plausibly, level-three moral principles which are applications of the categorical imperative. As will be seen later in this chapter, Act Deontology is open to serious criticism and, ultimately, it will be argued that Rule Deontology need not enter into our eventual position.

Duty-based ethics and the clauses of the UKCC Code of Conduct (1992)

One important point that may be made in relation to the duty-based perspective on nursing ethics is this: it seems reasonable to suggest that the clauses in the UKCC Code of Conduct (UKCC, 1992) attempt to set out the professional duties of the nurse. Otherwise, it would not be clear why nurses can be disciplined for practising in contravention of clauses in the

Code. Chadwick and Tadd describe this as a 'disciplinary function' of the Code (1992, p. 7).

Clause 1 of the Code states that registered nurses must, '[A]ct
always in such a manner as to promote and safeguard the
interests and the well-being of patients and clients' (UKCC,
1992). The similarity between this clause and the principle of
beneficence is significant. The clause makes clear that it is a
major part of a nurse's professional duty to promote the well-
being of patients and clients. As noted earlier, the principle of
beneficence generates moral obligations to act in ways which
promote the well-being of others.

Clause 2 states that a nurse must, '[E]nsure that no action or
omission on [his/her] part . . . is detrimental to the . . . safety of
patients and clients' (1992). According to this clause, nurses
must ensure that none of their actions or omissions expose
clients to risk of harm. It is significant that this sounds very
similar to the principle of nonmaleficence which, again as
noted earlier, generates obligations not to act in ways which
result in harms to others.

These parallels are highly suggestive. Further, it seems plausible to propose that the clauses in the UKCC code can be
understood as playing the role of level-two moral rules. Hence,
the clauses could be said to have their *moral foundation* in one
or more of the level-three principles described above. In this
way, the principle of beneficence can be said to constitute the
moral foundation of clause 1 of the UKCC Code, and the
principle of nonmaleficence can be said to constitute the moral
foundation of clause 2 of the Code. Before considering an
objection to this proposal, let us develop it a little further.

The proposal is that the clauses in the UKCC Code can be
construed as level-two moral rules which have as their moral
foundation one or more of the level-three principles. First,
recall that we referred previously to four level-two moral
rules: veracity, privacy, confidentiality, and fidelity. It is plain
that confidentiality is explicitly referred to in the UKCC Code
(clause 10).

Clause 9 makes mention of the 'privileged relationship'
which obtains between nurses and clients. It is reasonable to
construe this as closely related to the privacy rule – the clause
speaks of the 'privileged access allowed to [the client's] person,

property [and] residence . . . ' (UKCC, 1992). The characterisation of the privacy rule already discussed, frames that rule in terms of access to the client – as does clause 9 of the Code.

With regard to the fidelity rule, the Code makes no mention of the term 'fidelity', yet something very like the fidelity rule is presumed in the Code. We noted earlier that nurses implicitly promise not to practise negligently, and, perhaps, promise implicitly to practise in accord with the UKCC code. As noted earlier, nurses can be disciplined if they wilfully contravene clauses in the Code.

The fourth rule described earlier was that of veracity – crudely, that one should be truthful in one's dealings with clients and colleagues. This also seems implicit in the UKCC Code. For example, clause 5 states that nurses must 'work in an open and collaborative manner with patients, clients and their families' (1992). It is plausible to suppose that working in an 'open and collaborative' manner is possible only in a relationship in which truth-telling is the norm. Similarly, clause 6 obliges nurses to 'work in a collaborative and co-operative manner' with colleagues. Again, it plausible to assume that this is only possible in circumstances in which truth-telling is the norm.

So, it is evident that the four level-two moral rules identified by Beauchamp and Childress (1989) pervade the clauses of the UKCC Code (1992). Also, as noted above, in their employment of the framework, level-three moral principles provide the justification – or moral foundation – of level-two rules. This means that if we are to construe the clauses of the Code as level-two moral rules, it will turn out that they too have their moral foundation in level-three principles. We have seen how clauses 1 and 2 have their respective moral foundations in the principles of beneficence and nonmaleficence. The principle of respect for autonomy provides the moral foundation for clauses 5, 7 and 10: clause 5 obliges nurses to 'foster [the] independence' of clients; clause 7 states that nurses must 'recognise and respect the uniqueness and dignity of each . . . client'; and clause 10 concerns the obligation to respect confidential information.

The principle of justice might reasonably be said to underpin all the clauses, since it generates obligations to treat others fairly.

The relations between level-two rules and level-three principles will be clarified further in the next chapter when a more thorough account of the principles is presented. But, hopefully, the reader now has an understanding of the proposal which has just been made. The clauses of the UKCC Code have been construed as level-two moral rules; and it has been claimed that these have their moral foundation in one or more of the level-three principles described earlier (the principle of respect for autonomy, the principle of beneficence, the principle of non-maleficence and the principle of justice). This proposal has been supported by illustrations of the relations between certain clauses in the UKCC Code and level-three moral principles.

Arguments for the priority of level three of the framework

In this section it will be contended that it is level three of Beauchamp and Childress's framework for moral reasoning, as opposed to its other levels, which is the most relevant to moral deliberation in nursing ethics, and the following arguments in support of that claim will now be considered.

First, it is plain that level three is of greater moral importance than levels one and two. This is due simply to the fact that the 'direction' of justification appealed to in the framework is 'bottom up', so to speak: level-two moral rules justify level-one judgements. Hence, it is plain that level-three principles provide the justificatory anchors for level-two rules and, derivatively, for level-one judgements.

Second, two general types of level-four moral theories – Utilitarian and duty-based theories – were identified earlier. These, in turn, proved divisible into Act Utilitarianism and Rule Utilitarianism, and Act Deontology and Rule Deontology. Act Utilitarians and Act Deontologists base their decisions regarding what constitutes right or wrong action on considerations of each particular situation. But it is possible to level a number of criticisms at approaches which reject the adoption of general principles or rules which apply to relevantly similar sets of circumstances. For example, suppose it is claimed, either by an Act Utilitarian or an Act Deontologist, that an act of type A is morally right in circumstances of type C. It seems plain that theorists who make such a judgement must be committed to the view that acts of type A are morally right in all other circumstances of type C (cf. Hare, 1981; Beauchamp and Childress, 1989, p. 40).

For example, suppose acts of type A are acts of truth-telling, and circumstances of type C concern those in which a competent person requests information concerning his medical condition. It seems that Act Utilitarianism and Act Deontology must commit one to acting in the same way in all relevantly similar sets of circumstances. If act A maximises utility in one instance of C, surely it must do so in all instances of C. Similarly, when the position of the Act Deontologist is considered: if it is one's duty to tell the truth in one instance of circumstances of type C, it seems to follow that it is one's duty to do so in all circumstances of type C. So, the suggestion that Act Utilitarians and Act Deontologists simply consider one situation at a time is at least open to question. Decisions concerning what is right or wrong in one instance of a type of circumstance imply that the act theorists are obliged to act in the same types of ways in relevantly similar types of circumstances.

Further, against the Act Utilitarians and Act Deontologists it can be said that their proposal is of extremely limited use in practice. This follows since it requires persons to consider each situation anew, and to apply either the principle of utility or the categorical imperative to it. Seedhouse (1988, p. 94) points out that although many situations have aspects unique to them, it does seem possible to identify morally relevant similarities between situations. And, he suggests that the identification of common characteristics of types of situations can help to formulate general rules which can be applied in relevantly similar cases. Adoption of such rules (or principles) facilitates consistency in moral thinking, and, importantly, is intimately connected with fairness in the making of moral decisions. As noted earlier, put crudely, the principle of justice demands that equals be treated equally. Plausibly, this appears to require that we make consistent moral judgements in relevantly similar cases; and this in turn appears to require that some assessment is made to the effect that two situations are indeed relevantly similar or are not relevantly similar. This appears to conflict with the general approach to moral decision-making canvassed in Act Utilitarianism and Act Deontology.

The arguments presented so far in this section suggest that of the level-four theories identified above (Act Utilitarianism, Rule Utilitarianism, Act Deontology, and Rule Deontology), Act Utilitarianism and Act Deontology are open to serious objection.

Consider the following argument which is supposed to show that neither Rule Utilitarianism nor Rule Deontology are preferable to consideration of level-three principles when it comes to moral decision-making – specifically in nursing practice.

As discussed earlier in this chapter, Utilitarianism asserts that the rightness or the wrongness of an action essentially depends upon its outcome. From the perspective of a duty-based theory, on the other hand, the rightness or the wrongness of an act is essentially independent of its consequences; what matters is that the actor acts out of respect for moral duty. But it is not clear that either one of these options is desirable. Surely, when faced with a moral problem, one needs to consider both what is one's duty and what the consequences of one's actions are likely to be. This is especially the case in relation to moral problems faced by nurses. Given the links, argued for earlier, between the clauses in the UKCC Code of Conduct and morality, it is not clear that moral duty is, ultimately, detachable from professional duty. If correct, this indicates that, minimally, nurses are obliged to consider what is their duty when faced with particular moral problems in nursing practise – both moral and professional duty.

But, further, it is plausible to hold that nurses are also obliged to consider the consequences of their decisions about moral matters. For example, suppose a nurse undertakes a particular action, say, pressing a fire alarm. Suppose further that this is done out of respect for duty: the nurse believes there to be a fire on the ward, and so presses the alarm. The relevant professional duties here are those stated in clauses 1 and 2 of the UKCC Code (to promote the well-being of clients, and to act in such a way as to bring this about); and the relevant moral duties are those generated by the principles of beneficence and nonmaleficence. Evidently, the nurse presses the alarm because a consequence of not doing so is a high probability of harms to others. Plausibly, then, it may be held to be the case that the nurse is compelled to act out of respect for duty due to the necessity of acting in accord with the clauses in the UKCC Code, and due to the necessary connection between nursing actions and morality; and is compelled to consider the consequences of his or her actions in evaluating how to put duty into effect (how to make it the case that clients are protected from harm). So, in moral decision-making in the nursing context it seems reasonable to accept that it is necessary to consider both the consequences of one's actions and what it is one's duty to do. Indeed, further, it could be suggested that it is morally reprehensible not to consider the consequences of one's actions when making moral decisions. Rawls, for example, suggests that it is 'crazy', in moral thinking, not to consider the consequences of one's actions (quoted in Brown, 1986, p. 56).

So, it is being claimed here that it is necessary for nurses to consider both duties and consequences in their moral decision-making. To say otherwise seems, frankly, absurd. Another example to lend support to this point is the following: consider a psychiatric nurse who accedes to a request by a client to leave the ward, and that the nurse has good grounds to believe that the client is sufficiently mentally competent to leave the ward. From the moral perspective, the nurse acts out of consideration for the principle of respect for autonomy, and makes no attempt to physically prevent the client from leaving the ward (perhaps by invoking the holding power ascribed to nurses under the Mental Health Act, 1983). Suppose, further, that it then transpires that the client commits suicide and that the nurse is called upon to account for her decision. The nurse might argue that her decision was made to respect the wishes of a competent client and was grounded in respect for autonomy. Even if the nurse acts in that way (placing respect for autonomy over principle of nonmaleficence), the nurse should and would consider the consequences of the action. An investigating coroner might reasonably put to the nurse the question, 'Did you consider the possibility that the client might take their own life?' Presumably, the nurse, if professionally and morally competent, must have an answer to this question. Whether the nurse answers 'yes' or 'no' – and, conceivably, either of these answers may be acceptable depending upon the circumstances – it may be submitted that it would be almost contradictory for the nurse to make both of the following claims: (a) that she was acting professionally and morally, and (b) that she omitted to consider the consequences of her decision to accede to the client's competently expressed wish to leave the ward.

These considerations strongly suggest that in moral deliberations relating to moral problems which arise from nursing practice, it is necessary to consider both what is one's duty and to consider the consequences of one's actions.

It seems fair to conclude, then, that at level four of Beauchamp and Childress's moral framework, we should not retain an exclusive commitment either to Utilitarianism or to a Kantian duty-based morality but, rather, adopt the general stance in our moral decision-making that it is necessary to consider both consequences and duties.

In the light of the above arguments concerning level four of the framework, it will be proposed here that it is level three – that relating to moral principles – which is the most important level for our purposes. In brief, this is due to at least five reasons:

1. In contrast to the level-four theories, the level-three principles are easily applicable to the vast majority of moral problems faced by nurses. The principles provide a structure for the moral intuitions brought to moral problems by nurses. Consequently, consideration of moral problems through the lens of level-three principles ensures that practitioners consider the situation from a number of perspectives – the perspectives of each principle.

2. Second, overemphasis of the importance of level-four theories can promulgate or foster the view that there are clear solutions to moral problems: simply act in such a way as to maximise utility; or simply apply the categorical imperative. But this is too simplistic. Moral problems do not lend themselves to readily available answers thrown up by moral theories. It is surely preferable to consider the situation from a number of perspectives – those of the principles – rather than attempt to evaluate which course of action is

morally correct. Of course, a decision does have to be made; but it would seem preferable that such a decision emerge from consideration of various ways of viewing the situation, rather than, simply, implementing a particular level-four theory.

3. Further, from the author's experience of teaching nurses, it is evident that nurses themselves think the principles of level three easier to apply and more relevant to practice than the level-four theories. Given introductory outlines of the four principles, nurses begin to structure their moral thinking by reference to them.

4. Fourthly, as will be shown later, moral thinking at the level of principles does allow one to develop a coherent, well-motivated strategy by which to help to try to resolve moral dilemmas – given that these result from clashes between principles themselves.

5. Fifthly, nurses are bound by the professional obligations set out in the UKCC Code to respect the autonomy (for example, clause 5) and the individuality (clause 7) of clients. Also, as was seen earlier, it is evident that the principles of level three of the framework underlie many clauses in the UKCC Code (and the ANA Code – see Benjamin and Curtis [1986], pp. 179–81). So, plausibly, whether the ultimate moral justification for the principles is grounded in Utilitarian or duty-based considerations, nurses are required to engage in moral thinking at the level of principles simply to fulfil their professional obligations.

Merits of the principle-based approach

In this section, certain of the strengths and weaknesses of the principle-based approach to nursing ethics are considered. The principal merit of the approach, it would seem, is that it provides conceptual tools – the principles and theories of the approach – which may be employed to structure one's moral intuitions. Thus having learned the basic terminology of the principle-based approach one can consider moral problems 'through the lens', so to speak, of that approach (see, for example, Seedhouse, 1988).

For example, suppose a client requests details concerning the nature of medication prescribed for him. The nurse has to make a level-one moral judgment. Level-two moral rules referred to earlier include those of veracity, privacy, confidentiality, and fidelity. A quick consideration of these suggests that it is the veracity rule which is most relevant to the situation under discussion: that rule generates an obligation on the part of the nurse to give the information to the client. Of the principles, at least those of respect for autonomy, beneficence and nonmaleficence are pertinent here. Autonomy requires that the nurse provide the information to the client; beneficence generates an obligation to act in such a way as to promote the well-being of the client; and nonmaleficence generates an obligation not to act in ways which are likely to harm the client. Of our two theories, Utilitarianism demands that the nurse consider which course of action will lead to the generation of most good; and a duty-based view requires the nurse to apply the categorical imperative to determine what his or her moral duty is. A nurse who undertakes deliberations such as those just outlined can plausibly be said to have considered the situation from most relevant perspectives.

Further, it is evident that a nurse who bases a decision on deliberation is able to give an account in support of these actions. The nurse will have undergone a series of considerations, systematically, and applied these to the case in question. For example, the initial, unconsidered view may be that the client should not be given the information, perhaps on the grounds that the client might refuse the medication and will be harmed as a result. Suppose the nurse is asked to offer reasons why he acted in that way – say, withholding the information from the client. When this intuitive view is structured by the moral framework we have been discussing, the nurse should realise that such a decision is one according to which the obligations generated by the principle of beneficence are held to be more weighty than the obligations generated by the principle of respect for autonomy. The nurse might then seek to justify that mode of moral reasoning – perhaps by recruiting Utilitarian considerations.

Thus far, I have been relatively uncritical of the principle-based approach to nursing ethics. But there are at least three areas of controversy which may be mentioned here. First, there is the problem of which level of the framework, if any, is to have priority when it comes to applying it in practice. This particular issue is one which has been addressed in the present chapter. A second question concerns the weighting of the four principles which we have referred to so far. Are they each to be accorded the same moral 'weight', so to speak, so that in a conflict between moral principles we should be paralysed, and unsure how to act? Or, are some principles more weighty than others, so that in a conflict we may judge which principle carries most weight and hence which obligations are the more pressing? This question is one to be discussed in the next chapter following further consideration of the four principles. A third question is much more radical – this casts doubt on the legitimacy of the principle-based approach as a whole and champions an alternative, care-based approach to nursing ethics. Discussion of that debate is postponed until Chapter 5.

3 *The level-three principles*

The principle of respect for autonomy

The term 'autonomy' derives from a Greek word meaning 'self-governing' (see, for example, Beauchamp and Childress, 1989, p. 67). This gives some indication of what it means in the health care context. To say that clients have autonomy (or are autonomous), is to say that they have the capacity for self-government; in other words, that they are capable of making their own decisions about matters which concern their own futures.

As noted earlier, writers on health care ethics often refer to a 'Principle of Respect For Autonomy' (see, for example, Beauchamp and Childress, 1989.; Gillon, 1985). Again, as noted previously, what they mean is roughly this: we should respect the fact that persons have the capacity to reason and to make decisions which concern their own futures. Some commentators have suggested that the principle of respect for autonomy is the most fundamental of moral principles (cf. Downie and Calman, 1987, p. 50; also Harris, 1985; Benjamin and Curtis, 1986). What is claimed is that in the health care context, health workers should employ the principle of respect for autonomy in their dealings with clients. Further, the proposal is that if an autonomous decision made by a client is to be overruled by health care staff, then these same staff must be able to provide justifications in support of their action – the onus of justification lies with those who seek to overrule the autonomous decisions of others.

An example in which we might want to overrule a client's autonomous decision is a case where an informal client on a mental health ward makes a decision to leave the ward. A paper in the journal *Open Mind* (1991, pp. 7–10) is entitled 'Free to leave at any time?': the clear implication of the title is that although informal clients are legally free to leave, in practice that often turns out not to be the case. The writers of the article claim that almost 8000 requests to leave hospital made by informal clients in the year 1988–89 were refused. Such refusals indicate violations of the principle of respect for autonomy. The writers referred to an earlier claim that in such cases justification needs to be provided when autonomy is overruled.

What needs to be considered here is just what it is that is so special about the notion of autonomy that it should occupy such a central place in nursing and health care ethics.

Why autonomy?

As we have noted, many theorists writing in the area of health care ethics place great value on the principle of respect for autonomy. It might be worth considering why autonomy should be accorded such status – why should it be thought that overruling autonomy requires justification? Much hinges on this question since the reasons to be offered here contribute to a general claim that the obligations generated by the principle of respect for autonomy are the most weighty of the obligations generated by all the principles.

First, it can be noted that there is something slightly insulting about someone whom one meets and who simply presumes that one is not autonomous – perhaps the person treats one like a small child, making decisions on one's behalf which one is perfectly able to make oneself. Such a person is behaving paternalistically and one might justifiably feel offended at this. (Consider, for example, the title of the radio programme 'Does he take sugar?' – a programme for people with physical disabilities.)

If we as autonomous individuals object to being patronised, and if we feel uncomfortable when this happens, we may plausibly conclude that other people object to being patronised just as we do to it. We infer from what happens in our own case and generalise it to others: if we were in their position we would object to being patronised. When someone patronises us they are not respecting our autonomy, and many people object to being treated in that way. Seedhouse (1988, pp. 77–81) employs the term 'dwarfing'; when we patronise people we are dwarfing them – we inhibit them; the implication being that to behave in such a way as to dwarf them is morally objectionable. (Perhaps Seedhouse is guilty of 'sizeism' here.)

Second, it seems clear that autonomy is regarded as something of value at least in Western cultures, but perhaps also in all cultures. It is considered both desirable and psychologically healthy to be able to make up one's own mind, to be independent, and to be assertive when necessary (this, presumably, explains why some people attend assertiveness training classes). Further, it is considered undesirable to be excessively passive and unassertive. In short, it appears that we value independence, and regard excess passivity and compliance with the wishes of others as undesirable and perhaps even psychologically unhealthy. This indicates that it is regarded as both desirable and healthy to be autonomous.

In amplification of this last point, think of the following situation. You have applied for a job and you ask a friend to provide your prospective employer with a reference. Your friend offers you a choice of two references. The first states that you are able to think for yourself and use your initiative; the second states that you cannot think for yourself and that you lack initiative. Which reference would you prefer your friend to send? Presumably, none of us would wish the second reference to be sent!

Third, as seen in the discussion of Kantian ethics in the previous chapters, it is plausible to claim that the whole notion of morality is dependent upon regarding other people as autonomous agents – as persons who are responsible for their actions. It is common to think that someone can only act morally if they do so intentionally; that is, they act on the basis of a decision which they arrive at by the use of reason. So, if it is true that it is only possible to act morally if one is an autonomous person, this indicates how central the notion of autonomy is to morality. (Note how, in law, people are punished more severely if their crime is premeditated.)

Fourth, if one considers which crimes are regarded as the most grave, these appear to include murder, assault and theft. A diagnosis of why this is the case shows that these actions each involve serious violations of respect for autonomy. To murder someone is to thwart a lifetime of future autonomous actions and choices; to assault a person is to override that person's autonomous wish to decide what should happen to her body; and, to steal from a person is to remove the possibility of that person autonomously deciding what to do with whatever is stolen (see also Singer, 1993, p. 99, on this topic). It can be added that the proposed seriousness in morality of violations of autonomy is mirrored in law. The above crimes carry the most serious penalties.

Further, and fifthly, it can be pointed out that the point of many (all?) interventions by health care professionals is to enhance the capacity of clients to be autonomous (cf. Seed-house, 1988). For example, in the General Nursing context, suppose that a person needs to be admitted to hospital as a result of a badly broken leg. The person is able to make auton-omous decisions, but, due to the broken leg, is unable to put them into effect. The role of the health care team, here, is plainly to repair the relevant parts of the person's body so that the person is again able to act upon autonomous decisions. Similar examples can be constructed concerning other condi-tions – say, peritonitis – and relating to other kinds of nursing (for example, paediatric nursing and mental health nursing).

It can be added, further, on this point that the UKCC Code of Conduct (UKCC, 1992, clause 5) strongly indicates that it is the duty of the nurse to 'foster' the autonomy of patients and clients. Hence, nursing actions which induce avoidable depend-ence on health care professionals would appear to contravene clause 5 of the UKCC Code. Thus, actions such as feeding and dressing persons who can perform such tasks themselves seem to be in conflict with the UKCC Code. This point is especially pertinent in the context of working with persons who have learning disabilities, and in the nursing care of elderly persons. Also, the importance attached to autonomy seems reflected in law. Individuals are free to decide to reject even life-saving treatment. As Mason and McCall Smith state, 'Non-consensual medical treatment entitles the patient to sue for damages for the battery which is committed' (1994, p. 234). The above reasons, taken together, seem to indicate the enormous import-ance of the principle of respect for autonomy.

It might be objected that there are certain situations in nurs-ing where it is not possible to foster or develop the autonomy of clients. Perhaps contexts such as the nursing of dying clients might be thought to throw up such examples. But even here a plausible response to such an objection can be offered. It could be argued that dying clients should be enabled to make known any views they have concerning their death, and that these should be respected. Such views might concern issues such as resuscitation, organ donation, which relatives they would like to be informed, which religious figures sent for, and so on. Fostering the autonomy of dying clients, therefore, could be claimed to involve creating a context in which those clients are able to express their own views concerning their own death. Such persons would then be enabled to die their own deaths, so to speak, and not die in the way others think best for them.

So far, the discussion has been concerned with what autonomy is, and also why it is that ethicists might put such high regard on respecting autonomy. But it is also clear that there are occasions when it is overridden. This might happen if someone has a severe learning disability, or is in the acute phase of a mental health problem, or under the effects of drugs, or the advanced stages of senile dementia. So, clearly, there are occasions when, first, it is not possible to adhere to the principle of respect for autonomy (when someone is unconscious for example), and, second, there are occasions when one is justified in overriding the principle. Furthermore, the principle of respect for autonomy may be overridden when a person exercises autonomy in a way that will harm others (perhaps by assaulting them). Later, situations will be considered in which it could be thought justifiable to override the principle of respect for autonomy. Before doing so, though, it is necessary to consider the concept of competence.

Competence

Thus far in this book little mention has been made of the concept of competence. It is also fair to say that texts on nursing ethics generally do not attempt to distinguish the concepts of autonomy and competence (Melia 1989; Benjamin and Curtis 1986; Seedhouse 1988). But how do these concepts differ, and why is the concept of competence important?

It was pointed out earlier that, roughly, 'autonomy' can be taken to mean 'self-governing'. But, clearly, from the fact that one is autonomous and thus self-governing, it does not follow that one is necessarily competent. It may be suggested that whilst 'autonomy' refers to a general capacity of an individual, 'competence' refers to an ability to perform specific tasks (Beauchamp and Childress, 1989, p. 80). For example, nursing students may be autonomous in the sense of being able to make their own way to work, to decide which clothes to wear, to decide how much money to take to work and so on. Yet, in spite of these facts, a student might well not be competent to take a client's blood pressure – for example, if he or she had not yet been instructed in that procedure. Similarly, the student, though autonomous, may not be competent to perform any number of tasks – heart transplant operations, a service on a car, to give a lecture in nuclear physics and so on. So, it is clear that being autonomous is not a sufficient condition for being competent; but it does seem that it is a necessary condition. One can only perform a task competently if one is capable of deciding to do it.

The relevance of this distinction between autonomy and competence to nursing ethics is that in very many moral problems arising from nursing practice, the question of the competence of the client is absolutely crucial. For example, in the kind of case referred to in the *Open Mind* article mentioned earlier, it would be much easier to justify preventing a client from leaving the ward if the client is not able to make a competent decision to leave. Conversely, it would be much more difficult to justify standing in the way of the client's wish to leave the ward if the client's decision to leave is a competent one.

Another example of a moral issue in the nursing context which centrally concerns the concept of competence is the issue of informed consent. Clearly, to give one's informed consent to undergo a medical procedure one has to be mentally competent to make that decision – one has to be competent to perform the task of making the decision. So, it is evident that the concepts of autonomy and competence, though related, are distinct, and that each seems closely bound up with moral issues in nursing.

In continuing the discussion of competence, it will prove useful to say a little about factors which may affect a person's ability to make a competent choice, and to consider just how one might attempt to determine whether an individual is or is not competent. Factors which affect competence can be divided, very roughly, according to their physical or psychological nature.

Physical factors

Obvious physical factors which may affect a client's competence include drug intoxication and neuronal damage. A person who has consumed large amounts of drugs which affect the nervous system – for example alcohol or tranquillisers – may clearly have their capacity to reason impaired; as might a person who has sustained significant damage to their nervous system either due to physical trauma or disease.

It is important to bear in mind that a person has not lost the capacity to be autonomous until the parts of the nervous system necessary for rational thought are irreversibly destroyed (as is the case in humans in persistent vegetative states). Hence, individuals who are under the influence of drugs, or who suffer impairment of cognitive function due to transient neuronal damage, still possess the capacity to make autonomous choices. It is simply that at that time the person is not able to exercise that capacity due to the effects of the drugs or neuronal damage.

Psychological factors

With reference to psychological factors affecting competence, it is possible to identify anxiety, coercion and lack of information. If a client is extremely anxious, his capacity to make competent decisions is likely to be impaired. The point can be illustrated with an example – a case meeting to discuss whether a client is to be discharged from a psychiatric hospital. At the meeting are ten or twelve people: a consultant, medical students, nursing staff, nursing students, social workers, occupational therapists and so on. The consensus of the meeting is that the client is not yet ready for discharge. The client is then invited into the meeting, informed of the collective opinion and asked if he thinks it best that he stay in hospital a little longer. The client says 'Yes'.

Can the client's decision be regarded as a competent one? Many people find it difficult to speak in front of groups of other people – especially those composed of such powerful figures as consultants, nurses and social workers. It is not unlikely that the client will be so anxious in the situation just described that his main objective will not be to answer the question after consideration of relevant information, but simply to escape from the stressful situation. Such an anxiety-provoking situation as that just described is, to say the least, not conducive to the client making a competent decision. The example indicates how anxiety can adversely affect one's capacity to make competent decisions. Examples such as this indicate how important it is that nurses take their advocacy role seriously. One would hope that the nursing staff ensure that the client has expressed his real view, and point out to the other health care professionals the intimidating nature of the situation from the client's perspective.

It is also important to note that a person who 'chooses' one course of action as opposed to another due to coercion, cannot be said to have made a competent choice. Faulder (1985) points out that it is a feature of the logic of choosing that one has at least two courses of action open to one. The *Open Mind* article referred to earlier describes situations in which people who are in-patients in psychiatric hospitals may choose to discharge themselves. Upon voicing this choice, they are informed that if they try to do so they will be forcibly detained under the Mental Health Act (1983). A person who consequently omits to pursue their intended course of action, cannot be said to have made a competent decision to stay on the ward.

It was noted earlier that a clear distinction can be made between the notions of competence and autonomy. In explication of that distinction it was pointed out that a student nurse may be autonomous but not be competent, say, to take the blood pressure of a client – the student may not know how to use a sphygmomanometer. In this example, the student is autonomous but lacks the practical and theoretical knowledge necessary to take a client's blood pressure. Similarly, it was suggested that a student nurse may be autonomous but lack the competence to give a lecture on nuclear physics. In this case, the student lacks the knowledge to be able to give the lecture. Suppose this distinction is applied to examples relating to the taking of medication and the giving of informed consent. Given that it is evident that knowledge of specific information is necessary for a person to make a competent decision, it is plain that a person needs to know relevant information before he is in a position to make a competent decision to take or refuse medication. The expression 'relevant information', here, can be taken to include, minimally, the name of the drug being prescribed, the dosage, the benefits of taking the drug and also any possible harmful side effects. Just as the student nurse in our earlier example requires certain relevant information before being competent to use a sphygmomanometer, so clients require certain, relevant information before they can make competent decisions to take medication prescribed for them.

Consider now the relationship between competence and the giving of informed consent. Again, possession of certain information is necessary for one to make a competent decision. So, a client is only in a position to give informed consent to undergo a particular medical procedure when in possession of relevant information. Plausibly, this includes information relating to the nature of the proposed medical procedure, its anticipated benefits and any attendant risks associated with the procedure. It is especially important to stress that a client who simply signs a consent form without reading it, and who is not in possession of the information just described, cannot be said to have given informed consent. The client may have given their consent, but not their *informed consent* and it is the latter which is required from both legal and moral perspectives.

It may be added, here, that there seems to be a clear role for nursing staff in relation to the issue of informed consent. Nurses can perform an advocacy role by ensuring that clients actually do give informed consent when they sign consent forms.

Determining competence

As seen earlier, it may be the case that a client is not competent due to physical rather than purely psychological factors. For example, a client may have senile dementia to such an extent that he is frequently – perhaps permanently – in a disoriented state. Thus, it may be the case that even if attempts are made to furnish such a client with relevant information concerning a proposed treatment, that the client's state may be such that he or she is unable to understand it, and that this is due to neuronal degeneration. Similarly, a person with a severe mental health problem may be so confused or deluded as to be judged incompetent to consent to (or refuse to undergo) a particular treatment.

Further, consider that one is a nurse working with elderly clients, some of whom are extremely confused indeed. Suppose that one of the clients wishes to leave the ward, and it is feared that the client will come to some harm as a consequence of their confused state. From the moral perspective, much hinges on the question of the competence of the client. If he is competent to decide to leave the ward, it is much more difficult to justify trying to prevent the client from leaving the ward (since autonomous persons are generally not prevented from undertaking potentially harmful acts, especially if they make competent decisions to engage in such acts). If the client is not competent, then it is much easier to justify preventing such a client from leaving the ward (see the next chapter for an extended discussion of such cases). Moral problems such as these make acute the need for criteria of competence.

One set of such criteria has been put forward by Beauchamp and Childress (1989). Strictly speaking, they propose criteria of incompetence: if a person fails the relevant 'test' – for example, being unable to make a choice, as in item 1 below – then the person is not competent to make the relevant decision. The criteria listed by Beauchamp and Childress are as follows:

1. Inability to evidence a preference or choice;
2. Inability to understand one's situation or relevantly similar situations;
3. Inability to understand disclosed information;
4. Inability to give a reason;
5. Inability to give a rational reason;
6. Inability to give risk/benefit-related reasons (although some rational supporting reasons may be given);
7. Inability to reach a reasonable standard decision (as judged, for example, by a reasonable person standard). (Beauchamp and Childress, 1989, pp. 84–5; see also Buchanan and Brock, 1990.)

Note that these 'tests', are increasingly demanding; the criterion set out in item 6 is clearly more demanding than that set out in item 1. By item 6, a person is incompetent if he is unable to give reasons in support of and against (say) undertaking a particular course of action – perhaps discharging himself. But in item 1, a person only counts as incompetent if he is unable to indicate a preference. Thus, conceivably, a parrot could count as competent according to item 1, and not competent according to item 6 – provided the parrot could say 'yes' or 'no' when appropriately prompted.

Beauchamp and Childress state the criteria in the negative since they consider positive criteria of competence too problematic. However, in spite of their reservations, let us reconstrue their negative criteria positively:

1. Ability to evidence a preference or choice;
2. Ability to understand one's situation or relevantly similar situations;
3. Ability to understand disclosed information;
4. Ability to give a reason;
5. Ability to give a rational reason;
6. Ability to give risk/benefit-related reasons (although some rational supporting reasons may be given);
7. Ability to reach a reasonable standard decision (as judged, for example, by a reasonable person standard).

(with apologies to Beauchamp and Childress, 1989, pp. 84–5)

The character of the criteria still remains: test 1 is highly undemanding, whilst test 7 is much more demanding.

Test 1 Here, a person counts as competent if he or she is able to say 'yes' or 'no' (or shake or nod their head).

Test 2 In this case, a person is competent if he can understand his predicament and 'relevantly similar' situations. Presumably, some visible evidence would be required to determine whether or not a person understood his situation. Of course the expression 'understand his predicament' or 'situation' is far from clear. One way in which it might plausibly be construed would be to imply knowledge of one's location – spatial and temporal. Even this requires further clarification, since if someone is asked their location and answers 'Earth', then they are correct!

More appropriate criteria might reasonably require knowledge of (a) the present address of the person, and (b) a rough idea of the time and year. With respect to (a), this need not require that the person whose competence is in question be able to give the exact postal address, say, of the hospital or community home at which they are staying. But it does seem reasonable to require that the person knows the name of the town, and the name of the hospital or community home at which he or she is presently staying. With respect to (b) – temporal location – it seems unreasonable to require exact knowledge of this. At the time of writing this passage it is 10.30 am, 25 January 1994. But it is a struggle to recall the exact date (presuming that I am competent to judge the time). Also, it is common for people to make mistakes concerning the exact year – one might easily claim that it is 1993 and forget that it is 1994. For these reasons, it seems that only an approximate knowledge of one's temporal location should be expected of clients.

One might begin by asking the client if he knew the approximate time of day, then continue by asking the day, month and year. It seems excessively harsh to require exact knowledge of all these facts, but for it to be said that a person has a rough awareness of his temporal location one would expect that the person is not more than ten years out in answer to the question 'What year is it?', and is no more than five months out in answer to the question 'What month is it?' Whether or not the person needs to be asked which day of the week it is may plausibly depend upon other factors – say, whether the purpose of the client's trip out is relevant to the day of the week. If the person intends to use the Post Office and it is Sunday, there may be grounds to doubt that the person knows his temporal location.

In short, there is no simple means of determining whether a person knows his spatio-temporal location. But for it to be plausible that a person understands his situation, it can be expected that the person is able to offer a rough idea of his spatial location, and a rough idea of the year, month and time of day. These seem to be minimal requirements to be met by a person said to understand his situation.

In Beauchamp and Childress's statement of criteria for determining competence, they employ the phrase 'understand one's situation or relevantly similar situations' (1989). I have construed what it is to 'understand one's situation', perhaps, more broadly than they intend. Since, on the interpretation set out above, understanding one's situation amounts to knowledge of certain spatio-temporal facts, it is difficult to accommodate Beauchamp and Childress's other phrase 'or relevantly similar situations'. One possibility is that they intend 'understand one's situation', to mean something like 'understand the nature of one's [medical? or social?] condition'. Then, understanding relevantly similar situations would involve understanding of situations in which one, say, has a distinct illness but which creates similar problems – perhaps of psychological confusion or problems of mobility. Or, from the moral perspective, it may be that understanding one's situation involves something much more complex than understanding one's spatio-temporal location. For example, perhaps it means understanding that one is, say, at risk of possible harm if one pursues a certain plan of action (for example, going for a walk). Understanding relevantly similar situations then consists in understanding analogous cases – perhaps where the principle of respect for autonomy conflicts with those of beneficence, and/or nonmaleficence. It may be suspected that a combination of each construal of test 2 is the most appropriate here. But, it seems that the 'spatio-temporal' construal of test 2 is the more fundamental. A person competent to make the kind of judgement required by the second construal of test 2 must surely be able to satisfy the test in its spatio-temporal construal.

Test 3 This concerns the ability to understand disclosed information. Beauchamp and Childress's discussion of competence arises in the wider context of a discussion of informed consent. Hence, they point out that it is necessary that a person deemed capable of giving informed consent to undergo a medical procedure is able to understand information relating to that procedure. In the wider context, we may construe the test as relating to a client's capacity to understand information relating to, say, the risks of going for a lone walk (if the person suffers from confusion), or wishes not to take medication or wishes to discharge himself. For a person to make decisions of this nature competently, it is necessary that the person is able to understand information relevant to the decision (for example, the risks and benefits of pursuing the desired course of action).

Test 4 The ability to give a reason requires that the client be able to support an expressed preference with a reason. Suppose a person is asked 'Would you like to come to the shops?' A person who simply answers 'Yes' or 'No' has not given a reason. To return to the parrot referred to in the discussion of test 1, a parrot may be trained to answer 'Yes' or 'No' to questions, without the presence of any understanding on the parrot's part. Hence, it is plausible to suppose that it is necessary for a person to be able to offer a reason in support of undertaking a course of action, or undergoing some medical procedure. For example, suppose that a person upon being asked to sign a consent form to undergo ECT (electro-convulsive therapy) simply said 'Yes', and signed the form without reading it. That would not constitute evidence of the person's competence to sign. Again, suppose a person responds to the question described above ('Would you like to come to the shops?') with the answer 'Yes': test 4 requires that the person offers a reason. Perhaps he might answer 'Yes. I feel like some fresh air'.

Test 5 With respect to this test, a person is required to be able to 'give a rational reason' (1989, p. 85). This is more demanding than test 4 since it requires that the reason offered by the subject be a rational one. The difference being appealed to here can be exhibited thus: a person is asked why he or she does not wish to sign a consent form to undergo ECT. The reason offered is that the persons carrying out the procedure are Martians. This constitutes a reason and hence the person has met the criterion of test 4. But, of course, the person has not provided a rational reason in support of his utterance, and does not satisfy test 5. Alternatively, suppose a different person refuses to sign a consent form to undergo ECT. When asked to supply a reason, this person replies that not enough information has been provided concerning the nature of the treatment and its likelihood of success. Evidently, this is a rational reason for refusing to sign. In the second case, the reason offered is relevant to the refusal, but in the first case the reason offered seems to radically conflict with reality: the possibility that the team carrying out the ECT are Martians is so remote as to border on the absurd.

Test 6 This text is still more demanding and requires a subject to 'give risk/benefit-related reasons [for or against a particular decision or course of action]'. Let us reconsider the person in the last example who refused to sign a consent form to undergo ECT on the (rational) grounds of insufficient information to make a decision. Suppose the person is given the information and then considers the advantages (the benefits) of undergoing the treatment and then the disadvantages (the risks). Advantages might include the lack of toxicity of the treatment; disadvantages might include the discomfort usually experienced preceding and immediately after the treatment. Such a person qualifies as competent under the criterion of test 6.

Another example may involve a client who suffers from periods of confusion. Suppose the client is presently staying on a hospital ward for confused elderly people. The client states his intention to visit a friend who lives nearby, but the nursing staff are concerned that the client might become confused whilst off the ward and come to some harm. They express their worries to the client. The client says that he (or she) is aware of such risks, but is also aware of the benefits of taking a trip outside the ward independently. Such a client again meets the criterion set out in test 6.

Test 7 This final test is the most demanding, and requires that the person be able 'to reach a reasonable decision (as judged, for example, by a reasonable person standard)' (1989). This goes further than test 6 in that it requires the person to arrive at a decision which is regarded as that which a 'reasonable person' would make. Test 6 requires only that a person considers relevant risks and benefits, and offers no view on the nature of the eventual decision.

A difficulty, perhaps serious, with test 7 centres on the lack of clarity in the appeal to a 'reasonable person' standard of evaluation. Consider, again, the client wondering whether to undergo ECT. Suppose the client meets the criterion set out in test 6. It would seem that there are only three possible decisions that could be made: to refuse the treatment, to have the treatment, or to defer making a decision; and that any one of these would be reasonable. So in this example, it seems that test 7 is redundant. Provided the person considers the relevant risks and benefits – as required in test 6 – the person counts as competent.

What of our other client, the person who suffers periods of confusion but wishes to leave the ward to visit a friend? Again it seems, once the risks and benefits have been considered – as required in test 6 – there are only three options: to proceed with the visit alone, to reconsider, or not to go. As before, all three of these seem reasonable options.

It seems, then, in the light of consideration of these examples, that it is the criterion set out in test 6 which is of greatest importance in determinations of the competence of clients. It needs to be noted that the criteria are wholly independent of age-related considerations. A person may be competent to decide against life-saving treatment at age six, and not competent to do so at age 16 or 60. The application of this criterion is independent of the age of the person whose competence is being called into question.

One further point here: both Beauchamp and Childress (1989) and Buchanan and Brock (1990) suggest that criteria for determining competence should, to some extent, be decision-relative. That is to say, the criterion of competence the client is expected to satisfy is related to the seriousness of the decision being made. So, the less important the decision, the less demanding the criterion of competence required. And for important decisions correspondingly higher criteria of competence are required. For example, consider two situations. In the first, a person who is extremely confused is asked whether they would like a cup of tea or coffee. The person does not answer. The question is put differently: 'Would you like a cup of tea?' The person now answers 'Yes' (or for that matter, 'No'). The person meets the criterion of competence set out in test 1. Is there any point in trying to determine whether the person satisfies any of the more stringent criteria? Surely not – provided, of course, that nothing of importance hinges on the decision, for example that the tea contains arsenic or the person has a potentially fatal allergy to tea, and so on.

Consider now, though, cases in which people have more weighty decisions to make – such as in those examples recently discussed – decisions which could seriously affect an individual's safety or well-being. It seems entirely reasonable that more stringent criteria are required, so that the more important the decision, the more stringent the criterion of competence required. It is important to note, though, that as suggested above, the most demanding criterion is that of test 6. Considerations given above suggest that the criterion described in test 7 is redundant.

Considerable time has been spent, then, on the notions of autonomy and competence. The reason for this is that they are so crucial to what follows and in moral decision-making in nursing ethics that they require lengthy treatment. In fact, much more could be said in relation to either of these notions. However, let us now move on to consider a second level-three moral principle, that of beneficence.

The principle of beneficence

According to Beauchamp and Childress (1989, p. 194), the principle of beneficence generates 'an obligation to help others further their important and legitimate interests'. This is plausibly considered by Beauchamp and Childress to include core obligations to act in ways which will positively benefit others. The relevance of this moral principle to nursing ethics should be evident from considerations undertaken so far in this book. It was seen in Chapter 1 that all nursing actions can be regarded as having a moral dimension: all such actions are (or ought to be) for the ultimate benefit of patients and clients. Indeed, again as seen earlier, clause 1 of the UKCC Code (UKCC, 1992) states that nurses have a professional obligation to 'Act always in such a manner as to promote and safeguard the well-being and interests of patients and clients' (1992).

From the moral perspective, this can reasonably be interpreted as a statement to the effect that nurses are obliged to practise in accord with the obligations generated by the principle of beneficence.

It is a moot point whether members of the public and off-duty nurses are bound by obligations of beneficence, but it is certainly the case that nurses are so bound when they are officially on duty; this is made clear in the UKCC Code. Further, as we will be seeing later (Chapter 4), obligations of beneficence clash most often with obligations of respect for autonomy, to provide an extremely common variety of moral dilemmas in nursing practice.

The import of the term 'benefits' as it features in the principle of beneficence is worth briefly commenting on here. The benefits referred to can be understood, minimally, as physical and psychological benefits. Of course, it is unclear if these two types of benefits are, ultimately, separable. But it needs to be borne in mind that simply attending to physical problems can fall short of conferring benefits on clients. For example, it may be that the client's physical problems have a psychological cause – liver damage may be due to alcohol poisoning and the consumption of alcohol due to depression. So it is important to construe 'benefits' quite broadly here.

Further, there is a question as to the extent of the nurse's obligations of beneficence. The UKCC Code makes evident that nurses are obliged to have regard to the workloads on their colleagues, and to ensure that these are not so extensive as to constitute 'an abuse of the individual' (UKCC, 1984; cf. clause 13, UKCC, 1992). It seems, thus, that the obligations of beneficence to which nurses are subject extend to the well-being of colleagues. Given this, a further question arises: how are we to understand the term 'colleagues'? Does this cover only those people in one's immediate working environment – say, the ward one works on, or one's colleagues in a community team? Or do the beneficent obligations extend to all the nurses in the hospital or Trust within which one is employed? Perhaps the term 'sphere of responsibility' (UKCC, 1992) can help here. It may then be suggested that the nurse's obligations of beneficence extend only to those colleagues who work within the nurse's sphere of responsibility. This is certainly more realistic

– though not entirely without ambiguity even now (do nurses have a responsibility to all the members of their profession – and to society?).

Related to the last point is this. Just as the extent of the nurse's obligations of beneficence to colleagues may be unclear, so too is its extent to clients. For example, is the nurse equally responsible for the well-being of the clients on neighbouring wards as for the well-being of clients staying on her own ward? It seems plain that the nurse is most responsible for the well-being of those clients on her own ward (equivalently, her case-load). But, equally, if a nurse is aware of, say, gross malpractice on a neighbouring ward, then presumably, the nurse's obligations of beneficence would extend to the clients suffering due to that malpractice and she would have an obligation to try to protect those clients.

In short, it seems that the nurse's most weighty obligations of beneficence are to those colleagues and clients with whom she has closest professional practice and for whose well-being she is formally responsible (due to the Code of Conduct). But, given this, the nurse still has obligations of beneficence – less weighty than those just referred to – to colleagues and clients who may not fall within the nurse's immediate sphere of responsibility.

Two other points relating to the principle of beneficence are these. First, it is evident that other moral principles serve to constrain the obligations generated by this principle. (I am indebted to Gillon [1986] for the following way of characterising the relation between the principle of beneficence and other moral principles.)

For example, suppose a client expresses an intention to continue to smoke in spite of his having chronic lung disease. Obligations of beneficence generate obligations to promote well-being. Presumably, this can reasonably be taken to involve attempting to prevent the client from smoking – 'for his own good' as one might be tempted to say. So obligations of beneficence appear to motivate preventing the client from smoking – even if this is against his wishes. But obligations of beneficence clearly run up against, and conflict with, obligations to respect autonomy here. If the client wishes to smoke and his decision is a competent one, then the obligations generated by the principle of respect for autonomy indicate that the client's wishes should be respected. Here is a classical moral dilemma in nursing ethics (and health care ethics generally), which is generated by a clash between obligations stemming from different moral principles – in this case the principle of respect for autonomy and the principle of beneficence. This particular type of clash will receive extended discussion in the next chapter, and so will not be discussed further here.

The second concluding point concerning the principle of beneficence is this: actions which place obligations of beneficence above those to respect autonomy are describable as paternalistic actions. Roughly, they are actions for the good of someone else, but which conflict with that person's own wishes. In short, it can be said that the principle of beneficence serves to motivate paternalistic actions (a fuller discussion of this point follows in the next chapter).

The principle of nonmaleficence

The principle of nonmaleficence is the third level-three moral principle to be considered here. As noted previously, it can plausibly be taken to underlie clause 2 of the UKCC Code (UKCC, 1992) according to which a nurse should 'ensure that no action or omission . . . is detrimental to the . . . safety of . . . clients'. Also, apparently, Florence Nightingale said that hospitals should 'do the sick no harm' (quoted in Clarke, 1977, p. 17).

As with beneficence, there seem to be two fundamental ways in which one might harm others; namely physically and psychologically. Obvious forms of physical harms may result from assault and injury; obvious forms of psychological harms may follow from intimidation, threats and so on.

In their discussion of nonmaleficence, Beauchamp and Childress include as harms the 'thwarting, defeating or setting back of the interests of one party by the invasive actions of another party' (1989, p. 124). The term 'invasive' is not apparently intended to denote the kind of physical invasiveness of certain types of physical treatments, say, intravenous drip feeds, but is to be construed much more broadly. Hence, a nurse may be said to harm a client by omitting to provide the client with information concerning the toxic effects of medication prescribed for the client; or, by misleading a client about the success of a particular type of therapy, say, group psychotherapy. So it is evident that harm can be understood to encompass much more than mere physical harm.

It may be queried whether there is sufficient difference between the principles of nonmaleficence and beneficence to warrant the employment of two distinct principles with accompanying distinct sets of obligations (cf. Beauchamp and Childress, 1989, p. 121). But the different import of these two principles can be exemplified by reference to the UKCC Code. For example, as noted above, the principle of beneficence generates obligations to act in ways which promote the well-being of others. It was suggested that this principle provides the moral foundation of clause 1 of the UKCC Code. Suppose that instead of requiring nurses to promote the well-being of clients, the Code merely obliged nursing staff not to harm clients. Hence, clients entering hospital would not have their well-being promoted, but would merely not be harmed. Clearly, such a proposal seems absurd. Clients are referred to health care professionals to be made well, not simply to be protected from harm (though of course clients should expect this too). Obligations generated by beneficence seem much more demanding than those generated by nonmaleficence. The latter merely oblige one not to harm others whilst the former oblige one to benefit others.(Thus, beneficence would require us to help a needy, say homeless person, but nonmaleficence would require us merely not to harm such a person. See also Chapter 6 below on related issues.)

This account of the distinction between the obligations of nonmaleficence and those of beneficence can help to clarify the import of phrases such as 'appropriate [standards of] care' (clause 12) which figure in the UKCC Code. Given acceptance of the point that obligations of beneficence are more pertinent to health care than are obligations of nonmaleficence, it seems to follow that appropriate standards of care are those which foster the well-being of clients. Standards which merely provide a safe environment of care for clients can, thus, be shown not to constitute appropriate standards of care.

It may be said that in, say, caring for clients with terminal conditions, it is not possible to care for such clients in ways which promote their well-being – due to the nature of the client's condition. But it can be argued, first, that in such situations, the principle of respect for autonomy carries more weight and that care should be under the control of the client; and second, in the case of noncompetent clients, it may be said that care should be regulated by obligations of beneficence.

It has been noted here that the UKCC Code – and most (all?) other codes for health care professionals – asserts an obligation not to harm clients, yet routinely clients are subjected to harms. A person undergoing a physical operation such as an appendicectomy sustains physical harm when, say, the surgeon's scalpel cuts open the client's abdomen. Clients with mental health problems may be harmed by forcible admission to hospital or by taking toxic major tranquillisers. Of course there are numerous other examples of harms befalling clients as a planned consequence of regimes of health care; but clearly in many situations – especially in the case of, say, a competent client voluntarily acceding to an appendicectomy – such transgressions seem easily justifiable. In the case of a competent client, nonmaleficence may be justifiably overridden due to acceptance of the view that obligations to respect autonomy are weightier than those of nonmaleficence. So the obligations to act in ways requested by the client count for more than the obligations not to harm clients. Perhaps, even more obviously, it can be claimed that the benefits of undergoing the appendicectomy outweigh the harms which may befall the client if the operation is not performed.

More controversially, it may be claimed that nonmaleficence may justifiably be overridden in order to protect a person from avoidable harms. Perhaps compulsory immunisation programmes and compulsory detainment of persons under the Mental Health Act (1983) count as examples of such situations (we will consider cases such as these in detail later in Chapter 4). Still more controversially, it may be claimed that a person might justifiably be harmed in order to prevent harms befalling others. Compulsory immunisation programmes seem to count here, as may compulsorily detaining people who have a dangerous, easily transmissible disease. Also, it could be said that it is justifiable to harm (by restraining) a violent client in order to protect other clients and health care professionals. It is evident, then, that it is at least plausible that there are circumstances in which health care professionals may consider it justifiable to contravene their obligations of nonmaleficence.

Acts and omissions

Thus far, the discussion of nonmaleficence has focused on actions which involve intentional bodily movements the purpose of which is to bring about a specific, intended, state of affairs. The surgeon's action of cutting open a client's skin to perform an appendicectomy clearly counts as an action of this kind. But it is clearly possible to harm a person by virtue of what one omits to do – by omission – in contrast to harming a person by an intentional action – by commission. Clause 2 of the UKCC Code shows explicit appreciation of this point '[A nurse should] ensure that no action or omission on [his or her] part . . . is detrimental to the interests, condition or safety of patients and clients' (UKCC, 1992). Two examples of harming a person by omission are the following.

A person walking past a municipal fountain notices a small child drowning in it. The child is well within reach and could be pulled out with minimal effort. In spite of the easy accessibility of the child and the fact that the person understands that the child's life is in danger, a conscious decision is made to walk past and do nothing to help the drowning child.

A second example involves a nurse who deliberately omits to provide an unconscious client with medication without which the client will die (insulin or digoxin perhaps). It is to be supposed that the client is one for whom the nurse has clinical responsibility. The nurse simply omits to provide the prescribed drug in full knowledge of the consequences of such an omission.

Other examples include the following situations: allowing neonates to die by omitting to provide them with necessary nourishment (Kuhse and Singer, 1985); omitting to give a client information necessary to make an informed decision regarding a treatment option; or omitting to prevent harms befalling clients due to mistreatment of them by other health care professionals. Also, perhaps, omitting to take action to prevent avoidable suffering to the clients within one's 'sphere of responsibility' (UKCC, 1992).

So, it is clearly the case that we need to look a little further at the issue of harming others by omission and by commission. In fact, it has been asserted (and denied) that there is a moral difference between harming another by omission and harming another by commission. The view that there is such a moral difference stems from the acts and omissions doctrine, that:

> [In] certain contexts, failure to perform an act, with certain fore-seen bad consequences of that failure, is morally less bad than to perform a different act which has the identical foreseen bad consequences. (Glover, 1977, p. 92)

Thus, according to this doctrine, there is a morally significant difference between actively bringing about a state of affairs which harms another, and that state of affairs arising due to something one consciously omits to do. For example, suppose the prognosis of a very severely disabled neonate is extremely poor – the neonate is expected to survive for at most a month and during that time will experience great pain. Doctor A is in favour of bringing about the death of the neonate by administering a lethal injection. Doctor B, the infant's parents, and the rest of the health care team favour merely omitting to provide the infant with nourishment necessary for its survival. According to the acts and omissions doctrine, the 'treatment' regime favoured by Doctor B and the other is morally less bad than the regime put forward by Doctor A – even though the different regimes have the same intended outcome.

It is worth commenting that abandonment of the acts and omissions doctrine might be thought to lead to some uncomfortable conclusions. For example, we tend to believe that there is a moral difference between, say, acting in such a way as to blind a person – say by poking his eyes out – and merely failing to prevent the onset of blindness even though this could have been prevented. Charities commonly point out that a mere £10 donation can save a person's sight – typically a person in a poor country suffering from cataracts. Even though most of us reading this book could easily send such a donation, we omit to do so. Yet, we regard ourselves as morally distinct from a person who 'deliberately' causes the blindness of another person. If omissions are as morally reprehensible as commissions, there is no moral difference between ourselves and the person who 'deliberately' puts out the eyes of another. Perhaps fortunately, we do not need to possess a theoretical view on the acts and omissions doctrine – there are plausible arguments both in favour of it, and against it (see, for example, Singer, 1993; Glover, 1977; and Rachels, 1986).

What is important to note for our purposes is that one can be morally responsible for actions one omits to perform, in addition to acts one does perform. The question of equivalence in degrees of moral responsibility is a difficult one and perhaps it would detain us too long to discuss this at length. Suffice it to say that even if, in one case, bringing about harms by omission is morally speaking as bad as bringing about such harms by commission, it does not follow that in all cases harms brought about by omission are as morally bad as harms brought about by commission.

The principle of justice

This is the fourth and last of the level-three moral principles put forward by Beauchamp and Childress (1989). The term 'justice' may be said to have at least two senses (see, for example, Aristotle, *Nichomachean Ethics*, bk. V), the first concerns justice as desert, and the second concerns justice as fairness.

Justice as desert

The suggestion here is that if, say, a person works hard and saves money for the purposes of enjoying retirement, it is just that the person then does enjoy that retirement. The work that the person has put in and the sacrifices made, prompt people to judge that such a person deserves to have a happy retirement. It would be considered unjust, for example, if the pension scheme to which the person contributed became financially unstable and proved unable to provide the person with an appropriate pension. Similarly, if a student nurse studies hard during his or her education and is enthusiastic on placement experiences, it may be judged that they deserve to qualify.

Also, the notion of desert applies negatively, so to speak, in that one might deserve to be punished having performed some terrible crime. And further, in relation to health care, it may be said that a person 'deserves' not to be given scarce health care resources (transplant organs, for example) if the person has purposely pursued an unhealthy lifestyle.

Justice as fairness

In this case, the suggestion is that justice is done if people are treated fairly – where, roughly speaking, this involves treating equals equally. So, for example, suppose that a lecturer promises to give £5 to students who turn up for a particular lecture, but does not give all the students who turn up that amount of money. It may be said that the students who are not given the money are not being treated fairly.

Stated a little more precisely, the notion of justice as fairness can be said to imply that justice is done if equals are treated equally, and unequals treated unequally in proportion to relevant differences between them (see, for example, Aristotle, *Ethics*).

So, in the case of the students who miss out on the £5, it may be claimed that all the students present at the lecture are equally entitled to the money since they are all present; hence 'equals' are receiving equal treatment. Students absent from the lecture, thus, would not receive the £5 since they are not 'equal', in the relevant sense, to the students present at the lecture. In this sense, equals are treated equally and unequals treated unequally.

A different example is the following: suppose a parent of twins allows one twin to stay up after 9.00 p.m. but the other is made to go to bed at that time. The second twin may claim to have been treated unfairly.

Relevant characteristics

What is going on in these examples is that some judgement is being made concerning what is to count as a relevant characteristic or property of individuals, and a judgement made concerning the relationship of that characteristic to the action of the lecturer or the parent. So, in the lecturer example, since there is no relevant difference between the students present who receive the £5 windfall and those who do not, the latter group can claim to have been treated unjustly. Equivalently, the second twin may claim to have been dealt with unjustly due to there being no relevant difference between the twins.

The reader may be tempted to add further details. For example, in the lecturer case it may be conjectured that there is some difference between those students who do and those who do not receive the money. Perhaps the students who were given the money were particularly attentive and the lecturer wanted to reward them for this. If so, the action of the lecturer might now be regarded as just. This is because a relevant difference between those students who were given the money and those who were not has been posited. This difference constitutes the justification for distinguishing between the two sets of students: equals are being treated equally and unequals unequally. With respect to the twins example, it may be conjectured here that the second twin had misbehaved in some way and that this comprised the distinguishing characteristic between the twins.

So, in relation to the characterisation of justice as fairness offered above, evidently some judgement is required to be made concerning what is to count as a relevant characteristic in order that one is able to treat equals equally. One is required to put forward some criteria to warrant treating one group of students differently from the other group, and to warrant treating one twin differently from the other.

It is important to note that the actual formulation of the principle of justice (construed as an obligation to treat equals equally) is silent as far as the question 'What counts as a relevant characteristic?' is concerned. All the principle obliges us to do is to treat equals equally, regardless of how it is determined which properties of individuals are relevant to judging them as equals. Hence, treating equals equally requires some determination of the manner in which two individuals are equal. They may both be equal in the sense that they are humans, or that they are male, or that they are Brazilian, or that they turned up for a lecture, and so on.

These rough and intuitive reflections on an ordinary understanding of the notion of justice prompt a consideration of just
which properties of individuals are to be taken into account in
our evaluations of the fairness of particular actions (or policies,
or laws). Some characteristics of individuals seem clearly not to
be relevant in our moral judgements relating to justice. For
example, suppose the lecturer claimed that the money had
been distributed fairly. And, when asked what the basis or
criteria for distinguishing between the two groups of students
had been, he replies that it was the height of the students which
constituted the relevant characteristic: all and only those students over 5'10" were given the money.

From the moral perspective, one wants to ask what possible
relationship there could be between one's height and one's
entitlement to the £5. Imagine that a proposal of such a nature
was advanced in relation to the question of how to distribute
health care resources fairly. Suppose it is asserted that only
those over 5'10" are entitled to receive such resources. Plainly,
it would be absurd to judge that the height of the recipients was
a characteristic to be taken into account in the determination of
a person's entitlement to healthcare resources. (This would be
a form of 'heightism'.) Equally ridiculous characteristics could
be put forward (and rejected); suppose the health care resources are allocated only to those who are left-handed. Again, one
would say that distributing resources on the basis of such a
criterion would be wholly arbitrary from the moral perspective.

Hopefully, the reader can discern where these points are
leading. In judgements relating to the just distribution of health
care resources (or £5 notes, or privileges such as being allowed
to stay up after 9.00 p.m.), certain characteristics of potential
recipients of such resources seem relevant, and other characteristics do not. So far, it has been suggested that height and
being left-handed cannot plausibly be regarded as relevant
characteristics. What about a policy which distinguished between an individual's entitlement to health care resources on
the basis of characteristics such as age, gender or nationality?
Unless some kind of argument could be given to show that
these characteristics of individuals are ones which legitimately
affect their entitlement to health care resources, distinguishing
between them on the basis of age, gender or nationality

amounts to discriminating unfairly on the basis of characteristics which are not relevant from the moral perspective. Such a policy may be open, variously, to charges of ageism, sexism, or racism.

It is evident from our reflections so far that a necessary feature of justice is impartiality. The person making a just judgement, or who acts justly, is required not to favour individuals on the basis of considerations such as personal preference, or personal taste (see also Singer, 1993, ch. 2, for more on this issue).

Impartiality and the UKCC Code

An example from the nursing context may help here. Clause 7 of the UKCC Code states that nurses (etc.):

> . . . must recognise and respect the uniqueness and dignity of each patient and client, and respond to their need for care, irrespective of their ethnic origin, religious beliefs, personal attributes, the nature of their health problems or any other factor. (UKCC, 1992)

Recalling the characterisation of the principle of justice offered earlier, 'Treat equals equally . . .', this clause of the UKCC Code implies that *all* patients and clients are to be treated equally – the clause asserts a professional obligation to treat clients justly. So, the relevant characteristic of individuals which renders them recipients of the obligations of nurses is that the individual is a patient or client (again, for the sake of brevity the word 'client' will be used to apply to both patients and clients): nurses have obligations to treat all clients justly.

Suppose it is claimed that nurses have greater obligations to clients who are ill through no fault of their own, than to clients who are largely responsible for their own ill health. Such a claim would involve the assertion that a defensible distinction can be made between groups of clients – those who bear no responsibility for the onset of their ill health and those who do.

So, three types of properties of individuals are being appealed to. The first is that of simply being a client – call this 'property X'. The second is that of being a client whose ill health is not self-induced – call this 'property Y'. And the third is that of being a client whose ill health is self-induced – call this 'property Z'.

Clause 7 of the UKCC Code indicates that any individual who instantiates property X, is an individual to whom nurses have professional obligations. Given the relationship between nursing practice and ethics, which was discussed in Chapter 1, it may be concluded that clause 7 of the UKCC Code generates moral obligations to clients on the part of nurses. Further, these obligations seem to have their moral foundation in the principle of justice. This seems to be the case since that principle obliges those bound by it to treat equals equally; and clause 7 obliges nurses not to discriminate between groups of clients. As quoted above, the clause requires nursing staff to care equally well for clients regardless of their religious beliefs and so on.

Hence, it seems that the position espoused in the code asserts that insofar as an individual instantiates what we are calling property X, then nursing staff have obligations to treat that individual fairly. This entails not treating one client any more or less favourably than another. The hypothetical proposal advanced above, to the effect that individuals who bear most responsibility for their ill health should be regarded less favourably than other individuals, can thus be seen to involve a violation of clause 7 of the UKCC Code. By that clause, instantiation by individuals of properties Y or Z does not affect their entitlement to favourable treatment by nursing staff. Evidently, the point made with the help of the appeal to properties X, Y, and Z can be generalised: whichever properties of individuals are being posited as grounds for discriminating against those individuals (age, nationality, and so on), they cannot constitute legitimate grounds – at least if practice is to accord with clause 7 of the UKCC Code.

With regard to the point made earlier relating to certain properties of individuals which are relevant from the moral perspective, and those which are not, the following points may be made. It is evident that certain types of properties of individuals are ones which they have acquired by choice – or, at least, they are properties which the person acquiesces to voluntarily. Such properties might include being a supporter of Manchester United, being a footballer, being a father, being married, being a Conservative voter and so on. However, certain other types of properties of individuals seem not to be ones which individuals acquire with any degree of voluntariness. Examples here include, being human, being male (or female), being mortal, having white skin (or skin of any other colour), having brown eyes being a certain age, being born at a particular time, being born at a particular location (town, country or continent), and (perhaps) instantiation of any other property acquired nonvoluntarily.

In assessing which properties of individuals are most relevant from the moral perspective, it seems highly plausible to exclude those which the individual cannot help but instance or exemplify – being a certain, age, sex or nationality for example. Given acceptance of this view, a general position close to that apparently advocated in clause 7 of the UKCC Code seems to follow. When applied to the issue of how to distribute health care resources justly, the view implies that such resources should be distributed without regard for such properties of individuals. Hence, one's entitlement to a specific type of resource would be unaffected by one's age, sex and nationality. The plausibility of such a position is one we will consider at greater length in Chapter 4.

The proposal just advanced seems supported by the earlier point that autonomy is a necessary condition of morality. That claim seems to support a view in which it is held that properties of individuals acquired nonautonomously (characteristics not acquired as a result of an autonomous decision) should not count as morally relevant (that is, as grounds for benefiting or burdening an individual).

In recent times, two rival theories of justice have received much attention; these are the theories put forward by Rawls (1971) and by Nozick (1974). A brief outline of these two theories will now be provided and this will be followed in Chapter 4 by a consideration of the implications of the theories for the distribution of health care resources.

Rawls' theory

Rawls' theory identifies justice with fairness, and is generally characterised as an egalitarian theory. This is due to the fact that it seeks to distribute benefits and burdens equally among the members of a particular group – most obviously, among the members of societies. Rawls writes 'All social values . . . are to be distributed equally . . .' (Rawls, 1971, p. 62). It is also characterised as a contractarian theory (by Brown, 1986) – indeed, Rawls states that his theory owes much to the social contract theories put forward by Locke, Rousseau and Kant (Rawls, 1971, p. 11).

Clearly, a theorist who seeks to identify justice with fairness needs to clarify an understanding of the concept of fairness. By way of explicating this, Rawls describes a hypothetical 'original position' (1971, p. 17) in which individuals are able to characterise their view of what would constitute a just or fair set of social arrangements. Further, in making such a characterisation, these individuals do so behind a 'veil of ignorance', which is to say that they do not know in advance what their position in such a set of arrangements will be. Thus, for example, they will not know whether they are rich, poor, male, female, able-bodied, physically or mentally disabled, intelligent or otherwise, and so on.

Rawls suggests two principles which would be deemed fair: (a) '[A] principle of greatest equal liberty' (1971, p. 124) according to which 'each person is to have an equal right to the most extensive basic liberty compatible with a similar liberty for others' (1971, p. 60); and (b) 'The principle of (fair) equality of opportunity' (1971, p. 124), according to which 'positions and offices [are] open to all' (1971, p. 60). Within (b) is included 'The difference principle', according to which, 'social and economic inequalities are to be arranged so that they are . . . reasonably expected to be to everyone's advantage' (1971, p. 60).

With respect to the first principle, this is evidently a fairly straightforward endorsement of the principle of respect for autonomy. The principle asserts that the only restrictions on the exercise of one's autonomy stem from infringements of the autonomy of others (see, for example, Mill, 1861, p. 135). Not implausibly, Rawls supposes that such a principle will be chosen by subjects in the original position since they will choose not to have their own autonomy impinged upon.

As can be seen, the second principle divides into two parts. The first asserts equality of opportunity: positions in society will be open to any suitably equipped member of that society, and opportunities to acquire the appropriate equipment or qualifications will, again, be open to all. Evidently, then, social class, age, sex and so on, would not prove obstacles to candidacy for positions in society.

As for the second part of the (second) principle, inequalities in wealth and material possessions are permissible, but only insofar as the inequalities benefit the least well-off. Hence, such inequalities are legitimate only if the least wealthy are better-off in the presence of such inequalities than they would be in their absence.

As noted above, Rawls supposes that his principles will be acceptable to the subjects in the original position – behind the veil of ignorance. On the face of it, the supposition seems highly plausible. Given that the subjects do not know whether they will be rich, poor, physically disabled and so on, he supposes that they will opt for the set of arrangements in which their well-being will be protected in the worst set of circumstances (for example, if they have a severe disability which prevents them from obtaining employment).

In the next chapter, some of the ramifications of the adoption of a Rawlsian criterion of justice for the allocation of health care resources will be discussed; for now, the second of the theories mentioned above will be considered, that proposed by Nozick (1974).

Nozick's theory

As seen above, the starting point of Rawls' theory is a position in which no participant has any possessions or a clear idea of their natural abilities. In contrast to this, Nozick's theory begins from a point in which it is recognised that subjects do have possessions – described by Nozick as 'holdings' (1974, p. 150) – and natural abilities, and it is from such a starting point that he attempts to develop his theory.

Nozick proposes that 'the subject of justice in holdings consists of three major topics'. These are matters relating to: (a) '. . . the original acquisition of holdings'; (b) '. . . the transfer of holdings'; and (c) '. . . the rectification of injustice in holdings' (1974, p. 152). Hence, it is envisaged that there will be a principle of just acquisition of holdings, and a principle of just transfer of holdings. The third element serves to correct any transgressions of these principles of just acquisition and just transfer – say, by theft.

One of the merits of the theory noted by Nozick is that it is 'historical', which is to say that it takes into account how individuals come to possess their holdings. A person's holdings may have been inherited, or earned or justly acquired in some other way. Holdings are justly acquired if and only if they are acquired in a manner which does not contravene the principles of just acquisition or just transfer. This aspect of Nozick's theory accords with our intuitions regarding justice as 'desert' – at least in some ways; *pace* the application of the theory to inherited holdings (though, as noted, inherited holdings would be covered by the principle relating to the just transfer of them).

Nozick points out (1974, pp. 153–4) that other theories of justice seem not to take account of historical considerations in the way that his does. For example, a Utilitarian distribution of holdings would seem to consider at any one time the most equitable distribution of holdings at that time, as it accords, or fails to accord, with the principle of utility – regardless of events or patterns of distribution prior to that time. The justice or injustice of the distribution at a specific time would be wholly independent of historical considerations.

Similarly, egalitarian theories (such as that proposed by Rawls), when considered from Nozick's perspective, may be charged with ignoring relevant historical factors. For example as noted earlier, Rawls' theory asserts a 'difference principle' according to which any inequalities in holdings between members of a society are justified only if they benefit the least well-off. Thus, Rawls' theory places the 'end result', so to speak, of just distribution of holdings across a society above an individual's own historical claims to retain possession of those holdings. Thus, in Rawls' view, justice demands that holdings acquired, for example, by hard-working members of a society could justifiably be redistributed to less well-off members (as in taxation). Such a redistribution would only be legitimate in Nozick's account, if it had the consent of those with the holdings in the first place. Hence, if the principle of justice as applied in that society is construed in Nozick's terms, taxes due to be distributed to the least well-off can only be allocated to that group with the consent of individual, rich members of the society. In fact, Nozick writes, 'Taxation of earnings from labour is on a par with forced labour' (1974, p. 169). Also, with reference to the expression 'end result' as used above, it should be said that Nozick contrasts 'end-result' principles of justice with his own 'historical' principles (1974, p. 155).

So far, then, a brief description has been given of the main components of Nozick's theory, a motivation for it, and a consequence of its adoption. Those unpersuaded of the merits of the theory are issued with a challenge by Nozick. Critics are invited to apply their own favoured theory of just distribution of holdings to an example supplied by Nozick; call this favoured schema of just distribution, D1. (D1 may be a distribution in accord with Rawlsian criteria, or according to Utilitarian criteria, for example) When this is done, he supposes, the theory of justice which most accords with the reader's intuitions concerning justice will be Nozick's own. The example is referred to as the 'Wilt Chamberlain' argument (by Honderich, 1979, p. 94).

Nozick's Wilt Chamberlain example

Nozick invites us to suppose that Wilt Chamberlain is a great basketball player and that when he plays home games, attendances are above average. Further, suppose that Chamberlain's crowd-pulling capacities are recognised and that he negotiates a contract in which '. . . twenty-five cents from the price of admission goes to him' (1974, p. 161). Nozick continues:

> Let us suppose that in one season one million persons attend his home games, and Wilt Chamberlain ends up with $250,000, a much larger sum than the average income and larger even than anyone else has. Is he entitled to this income? Is this . . . distribution [of holdings] unjust?

Call the resulting pattern of distribution D2 – that in which Wilt Chamberlain receives the large sum – and note that this results from our favoured pattern of distribution, D1. Also, bear in mind, of course, the fact that those who attend the games do so voluntarily, and autonomously choose to give their 25 cents to Wilt Chamberlain having previously been made aware of the details of his contract. Nozick's conclusion is that Wilt Chamberlain is entitled to the sum of money accrued, and that it is a just distribution of holdings. Further, it seems to be a distribution which accords with our intuitions concerning acquisition and transfer. The money acquired by Chamberlain is voluntarily given to him by parties concerned and so, it seems, must accord with any principles relating to the just transfer of holdings. Since D2 results from D1, and D2 is regarded as just, then D2 must also be a just distribution. (Nozick writes 'If D1 was a just distribution, and people voluntarily moved from it to D2 . . . isn't D2 also just?')

However, a quite serious objection may be levelled at Nozick's theory, and this centres on the intuitions appealed to in the Wilt Chamberlain example. For example, suppose that Chamberlain earns £200000 through the money-making scheme described above. Suppose, further, that a person who has such severe disabilities that they are unable to work and with no earning power is, as Kymlicka puts it, 'on the verge of starvation' (Kymlicka, 1990, p. 100). In Nozick's theory, there is no obligation on the part of wealthy citizens to aid the poor – even starving – citizens. Kymlicka suggests: 'Surely our intuitions . . . tell us that we can tax Chamberlain's income to prevent that starvation'. In Nozick's theory, those in possession of holdings can dispose of them in any way they choose, even if this results in the kind of situation just described. Hence, the suggestion here is that Nozick's theory has an implication which conflicts so greatly with intuitions concerning justice that it is rendered implausible. Also, it may be said that those who share the intuition appealed to by Kymlicka may take it to lend support to Rawls' theory. This is due to the role of the Difference Principle according to which, it may be recalled, great inequalities in material wealth are permissible only if the less well-off are better-off in their presence.

What can be taken from this brief outline of the two theories of justice, is that two fundamentally different views regarding what constitutes justice can be well-supported. Further, when the two theories are applied to questions of resource allocation, they throw up different approaches. A Rawlsian view, for example, seems congenial to a schema of resource allocation which considers the health of all citizens. For, in Rawls's hypothetical original position the participants will be ignorant of their own health status and may be presumed to take this into account in their views concerning allocations of health care resources.

Thus, the Rawlsian view can be contrasted with Nozick's line. In this, roughly, the good of all citizens is not necessarily a matter of concern to the individual; the individual's interests carry more weight than the interests of other members of society. Nozick's theory seems more congenial to a schema of distribution of health care resources in which it is up to individuals themselves to arrange their own health care needs (presumably by insurance).

Thus, applied to health care, a Rawlsian approach, it seems, would seek to maintain the health of all the members of the state, and, hence, to ensure that the institutional structures necessary to implement that aim are in place (community care structures, hospitals, dental care, eye care, health information and promotion and so on). A Nozickian approach to health care provision would very much leave it to the individual to arrange for their own health care needs to be met. Market forces would compete to provide the structures necessary to meet those needs. It should be said that it seems likely that nurses and other groups of health care professionals would be more likely to embrace a Rawlsian line rather than a position close to that put forward by Nozick. This is because in the Rawlsian position it seems more likely that the state apparatus necessary to implement health care would be in place; and, one imagines, this would appeal to those citizens who have an interest in the well-being of all the members of a state.

Conclusion

Having considered all four principles, it may be claimed that the principle of respect for autonomy is the most weighty. This general position seems motivated by the discussion of autonomy at the beginning of this chapter. There, it was claimed that the importance of autonomy can be derived from a number of considerations: for example, that many – perhaps most – people find paternalism objectionable; that autonomy is highly valued and its absence considered psychologically unhealthy; that autonomy seems a necessary condition of morality; that the most serious crimes (murder, rape, theft) seem so because they involve profound violations of autonomy; and that the point of health care, it seems, is to restore and foster autonomy. Further, as seen, the legal position in the UK (and elsewhere) appears to reflect the weight accorded here to the principle of respect for autonomy. This is evidenced by the fact that autonomous persons are legally able to refuse even life-saving treatments, and that the consent of competent clients is legally required before treatment is permissible (except emergency treatment, of course, where the wishes of the client are not known).

These points indicate that respect for autonomy is weightier than the principles of beneficence or nonmaleficence since competent decisions to refuse to submit to beneficent or nonmaleficent actions are generally respected. With regard to the principle of justice, this functions as a constraint on autonomy, as for example when the exercise of autonomy involves violations of the autonomous wishes of others. Also, justice is invoked when it is not possible to respect autonomy; for example, as may be the case in matters of resource allocation, justice is invoked solely because it is not possible to respect the autonomous wishes of those who require access to resources. Hence, the position outlined in this chapter can, for obvious reasons, be described as an 'autonomy-weighted' principle-based approach. Problems with this approach are discussed in Chapter 5.

4 *Conflicts between principles*

In the last chapter, each of the level-three moral principles which figure in Beauchamp and Childress's principle-based approach was considered. Given understanding of the nature of the obligations generated by these principles, we now move to consider examples of moral dilemmas which arise due to clashes between moral principles. Specifically, we consider clashes between the principle of respect for autonomy, and the principles of beneficence, nonmaleficence and justice.

Respect for autonomy in conflict with beneficence and nonmaleficence

A great many of the moral problems faced by nurses stem from conflicts between obligations generated by the principle of respect for autonomy on the one hand, and obligations generated by the principles of nonmaleficence and beneficence on the other.

Truth-telling

For example, consider truth-telling. Suppose a client has a terminal condition and that the health care team believe that informing the client about the nature of his condition will make him depressed and merely add to his level of suffering. Further, it may even be the case that the client's relatives have been informed about the nature of his condition and that they have requested that the client not be told. This case appears to present a clear clash between the principle of respect for autonomy and the principle of nonmaleficence.

It may be asked what the relation is between truth-telling and the principle of respect for autonomy. But it can be shown that there is a clear link between these notions and, hence, that the level-two rule of veracity has its moral foundation in the level-three principle of respect for autonomy. (It may be re-called that the veracity rule generates obligations to be truthful – see Chapter 2 of this volume.) For example, Rowson writes:

> [If] someone lies to you, he is reducing your capacity to under-stand your surroundings; and since this capacity is a valuable part of you as a person, he is thus failing to respect you as a person . . . (1990, p. 19)

Hence, the suggestion here is that as an autonomous agent one needs information in order to maximally exercise one's free-dom of choice. For example, suppose you know that I am a keen supporter of Wycombe Wanderers and that I am unaware of the fact that they are playing tonight. You, however, know that they are playing tonight and you deliberately keep this information from me – information it is plausible to suppose that I would like to be given. In purposely keeping this infor-mation from me, you reduce the number of choices I recognise as being available to me and thereby inhibit my autonomy.

DNR ('do not resuscitate') decisions

Similarly, consider situations in which a competent client is not involved in discussions concerning her resuscitation status. The motivations for not involving the client may be of two general types.

First, the client may be excluded from the decision-making process on the grounds that such decisions are medical rather than moral. But this can quickly be shown to be objectionable. Recall from Chapter 1 above, that the concerns of applied ethics include situations or actions which harm or benefit persons. Since a decision not to resuscitate a person will plainly either harm or benefit that person, such a decision necessarily has a moral aspect. Further, as we saw in Chapter 3 during the discussion of nonmaleficence, it is possible to bring about a person's death by omission, as opposed to commission. It may be that a DNR order is placed on a client to prevent the client from further suffering. Deaths brought about in consideration of the interests of a person are plausibly described as a conse-quence of acts of euthanasia (deaths brought about against a

persons wishes and for no benefit to the person could reasonably be described as acts of murder). One form of euthanasia
is passive euthanasia, which involves bringing about a person's death by omission. Evidently, then, DNR decisions implement passive euthanasia since they are decisions to bring about
the death of an individual by omission (the omission to act in
ways which will prolong the person's life). So, it is highly
plausible to assert that DNR decisions have a moral component
for the reasons just given. Plainly, medical facts may be relevant to a moral decision – for example, if a person has only a
few days to live which will inevitably be spent in great pain.
But the point remains that decisions not to resuscitate clients
(or, indeed, decisions to resuscitate them) inescapably have a
moral component (see, for example, Yarling and McElmurry,
1983).

The second type of motivation for not involving clients in
DNR decisions, arises from consideration of the possible harms
or psychological distress which clients might suffer (but see
Robertson, 1993). The view here seems to be that obligations of
nonmaleficence are so great as to outweigh those to respect the
autonomy of clients (see Loehy, 1991).

We have seen two types of issues, then, arising from nursing
practice, in which there is a conflict between the principle of
respect for autonomy on the one hand, and those of beneficence and nonmaleficence on the other. In fact, there are
countless other types of situations in which this type of conflict
occurs. A brief list might include the following:

- Asking clients to get out of bed or to move when they do not
  wish to;
- Asking clients to return to a ward when they do not wish to;
- Asking clients to take medication when they do not wish to;
- Trying to prevent a client from leaving a ward;
- Entering a client's house without the client's permission;
- Moving a client (say, a client with a severe physical dis-
  ability) without seeking the client's views on the matter;
- Feeding or giving medication to a client against that client's
  wishes;
- Trying to wash a client without the client's permission, or
  against the client's wishes;

- Treating a client against that client's wishes;
- Trying to prevent a client from committing suicide; etc.

It is perhaps no exaggeration to say that a very significant proportion of the moral problems faced by nurses in their interactions with psychologically competent clients arise from conflicts between the principle of respect for autonomy and those of beneficence and nonmaleficence.

Autonomy and paternalism

Put roughly, acts which are intended to benefit, or prevent harm befalling another person, but are not at the request of that person, can be described as paternalistic acts. Benjamin and Curtis (1986) favour the term 'parentalism', as opposed to 'paternalism' which may be open to the charge of sexism: clearly female parents may also act paternalistically, and parentalism seems the more accurate term here. In spite of this, I will continue to use the term 'paternalism', since 'parentalism' seems not to be in common usage and may cause confusion. Benjamin and Curtis characterise paternalistic acts rather memorably as acts in which:

> The nurse [or other health care professional] will claim to be acting *on the behalf*, although *not at the behest*, of the patient [or client]. (1986, p. 53)

Hence, suppose a nurse intentionally disregards a client's expressed wishes not to receive pressure-area care – the client finds the procedure causes discomfort and is a little painful. The nurse continues to turn the client over, however, and give the pressure-area care in spite of what the client says.

The nurse in such a situation seems to be acting in a way which satisfies Benjamin and Curtis's characterisation: the nurse is, in her view, acting on behalf of the client though not at the behest of the client – the opposite in fact.

A parallel analysis can be given for all the types of situations listed a few paragraphs earlier. The nurse wants to act in accord with what he or she thinks to be in the client's best interests, in spite of the client's own views on the matter. It is, perhaps, worth noting that the term 'paternalism' is intended to suggest the adoption of a parental, protective attitude towards others – in our case, clients or other health care colleagues. Also, it should be recalled that paternalistic actions are motivated by obligations of beneficence and nonmaleficence.

It needs to be stressed that paternalistic actions are not objectionable *per se*. Indeed, as just noted, such actions may be motivated by adherence to respectable moral principles. However, given the apparent importance or moral weight accorded to the principle of respect for autonomy in this discussion, it may be claimed that any actions which seek to override the autonomy of another moral agent stand in need of justification.

It is important to emphasise the position just described: a theoretical stance within nursing ethics being proposed here is that in nursing practice, actions which seek to override the autonomy of a client stand in need of justification. Hence, the mere fact that an action is perceived by nurses (or other health care professionals) to be for the benefit of a client, is not sufficient justification for adoption of that course of action. Thus, it is being put forward here that paternalistic actions stand in need of moral justification.

One point of clarification is needed before continuing. Recall that for Benjamin and Curtis an action is paternalistic if it is on someone's behalf but not at that person's behest. In each of the examples of paternalistic actions which were offered earlier, the client was conceived to be autonomous; more specifically, the person was conceived to be conscious, rational and able to make a decision. In cases of this nature, obligations of beneficence and nonmaleficence clearly conflict with obligations to respect autonomy. But, consider cases in which, say, a person is unconscious and where the person has expressed no view whatsoever with regard to preferences concerning health care (the person has not left a living will, for example).

In cases such as these, there is no evident conflict with the autonomy of the unconscious person since that person is not able to express any preferences; and, we are supposing that the person has not hitherto expressed any preferences regarding health care options. Actions intended to benefit such an unconscious person apparently qualify as paternalistic on Benjamin and Curtis's criterion, since they are for the benefit of the unconscious person but not at their behest. This quite broad characterisation of paternalistic acts is in agreement with much modern usage, and so it will be followed here. (See, for example, Beauchamp and Childress, 1989, p. 214, '... "paternalistic interventions" in our usage do not necessarily override autonomy'; and Dworkin, 1971, referred to in Culver and Gert, 1982, p. 127.)

It should be clear, then, that paternalistic acts here are to be construed quite broadly to include acts which are for the benefit of another person. It seems uncontroversial to point out that acts which benefit persons who are unable to express a view on the matter – unable to express any preferences – are fairly easy to justify from the moral perspective. This follows from our earlier points regarding the obligations of beneficence and nonmaleficence which bind nurses. As before, it is presumed that the client has expressed no prior views regarding preferences for treatment options.

Much more controversial moral problems arise from two kinds of cases. First, those in which an autonomous client makes a competent decision to pursue a course of action which, in the view of the nurse, will not benefit the client and may be harmful to the client. Examples of such situations include cases where clients refuse medication, refuse to get out of bed, refuse pressure-area care, seek early discharge, take harmful drugs, express intentions to commit suicide and so on. Moral problems of this nature involve conflicts between obligations of respect for autonomy and those of beneficence and nonmaleficence.

The second kind of cases include situations in which it is difficult to determine whether or not the client is, in fact, competent to make a decision to pursue a course of action which, in the view of the nurse, will not benefit the client and may be harmful to the client. The examples offered in the last paragraph can be cited once more here. The areas of nursing in which situations of this nature arise most frequently, it can be supposed, include nursing children, nursing elderly clients and in the mental health setting. Often in those areas it is extremely difficult to determine whether a client is indeed competent to make a particular decision.

Given acceptance of our earlier claims regarding the importance of respecting the autonomy of clients, it would seem to
follow that in straightforward clashes between that principle
and those of beneficence and nonmaleficence, that obligations
to respect autonomy win out. Though, as will shortly be seen,
there are serious problem cases, especially with regard to suicidal clients.

If that theoretical stance is accepted, it would follow, further,
that the greater the degree of autonomy and competence of
a client, the more difficult it is to justify acting paternalistically
– that is, acting in that person's interests as they are conceived
by health care professionals, as opposed to how they are
conceived by the client. Having made these points, let us continue.

The question which needs to be addressed is this: can there be
paternalistic interventions which are morally justified given
both: (a) the earlier claims regarding the moral weight attached
to autonomy, and (b) given that our concern is specifically with
moral problems in which the client at least appears to be both
autonomous and competent?

Justifying paternalistic interventions

Benjamin and Curtis (1986) offer three necessary conditions
which have to be met in order to justify a paternalistic intervention. They claim that:

> An act of parentalism . . . [is] justified if and only if:
> 1. the subject is, under the circumstances, irretrievably ignorant of
> relevant information, or his or her capacity for rational reflection
> is significantly impaired (the autonomy condition);
> 2. the subject is likely to be significantly harmed unless interfered
> with (the harm condition); and
> 3. it is reasonable to assume that the subject will, at a later time,
> with greater reflection, ratify the decision to interfere by consent-
> ing to it (the ratification condition). (1986, p. 57)

Hence, for Benjamin and Curtis, three conditions must be satisfied in order for a paternalistic action to be morally justified.
These will be discussed in turn.

The autonomy condition

If a subject is aware of 'relevant information' and if the subject is able to reason – capable of 'rational reflection' – then paternalistic interventions will not be justifiable. In short, if a client is competent to make a decision to pursue a particular course of action, it is not justifiable to prevent him.

It should be stressed that there are no obligations to respect autonomy if a person is exercising that autonomy in a way which will harm others (see, for example, Mill, 1861, p. 135). If a person enters my room with a gun and expresses an intention to shoot me, I am not obliged simply to respect his autonomous wish to do so! Obligations to respect autonomy do not apply when a person seeks to violate the autonomy of other moral agents.

In Benjamin and Curtis's view, for a paternalistic intervention to be justified, it is necessary that the client is not autonomous – more specifically, that the client is not competent.

The harm condition

By this, for a paternalistic intervention to be justified it is necessary that the client is open to high risk of 'significant harm'. If no harm is likely to befall the client, then a paternalistic intervention cannot be justified. Perhaps more seriously, the mere fact that a course of action recommended by a health care professional is likely to benefit a client is not taken to be a sufficient justification for a paternalistic intervention. This position sits well with our earlier points regarding the relative moral weight attached to autonomy and beneficence.

One immediate difficulty with the harm condition appears to be raised by the term 'significant harm'. It seems plausible to suppose that, say, a course of action which will lead to serious injury (loss of a limb, for example), will count as significant harm. Further, it is possible to identify a class of harms which may be described as psychological. Severe depression, schizophrenia and other mental health problems which involve distress to their sufferers all seem to be relevant here. Benjamin and Curtis offer only the example of cigarette smoking as an activity which runs a high risk of significant harm (1986, p. 60).

In spite of difficulties concerning its application, the term 'significant harm' of Benjamin and Curtis might still prove to be worth taking seriously. This, once more, is due to the view that autonomy carries more moral weight than nonmaleficence. Hence, it is evident that persons capable of competent decisions are not prevented from undertaking activities which involve a high risk of significant harm. Examples of such activities include smoking, heavy alcohol consumption, excessive consumption of unhealthy foodstuffs, cycling, mountaineering, motor racing, motor cycling, boxing and so on. Clearly, in the prevailing moral climate (in Western cultures), autonomous persons (specifically those over the age of 18) are not prevented from undertaking harmful courses of action. To accept this position for persons outside the health care context, and to deny it for clients of health care professionals, would seem to constitute unprincipled discrimination against the latter group of individuals.

To a large extent, then, any worries one has over the extent of the application of the term 'significant harm' can be put to one side in a substantial class of cases. Specifically, cases in which autonomous individuals make competent decisions to engage in types of actions which are harmful to them and to them alone. Indeed, such a position is reflected in the law (see Chapter 3 above). Competent adults are entitled to refuse even life-saving treatment, and to treat them against their wishes constitutes criminal assault (Mason and McCall Smith, 1994, p. 234).

So, it seems reasonable to suppose that we may accept Benjamin and Curtis's second condition, the harm condition, according to which, for a paternalistic intervention to be justified, it is necessary that the client will come to significant harm unless intervention takes place. It is important to note that this condition is not a sufficient condition for the justification of paternalistic acts. This is due to the fact that if a client fails to satisfy the autonomy condition – if he or she is both autonomous and competent – then the fact that that condition is not satisfied indicates that the paternalistic intervention is not justified (since, in effect, Benjamin and Curtis require that a person is not competent before a paternalistic intervention may be enacted – see for example, 1986, p. 57).

The ratification condition
This third condition put forward by Benjamin and Curtis may be explicated by reference to examples of the following kind.

In the mental health context, it is sometimes the case that clients refuse medication and do so during phases of acute illness. For example, suppose such a client refuses medication on the grounds that the medication was manufactured by 'devils'. Suppose, further, that the client is given medication against their wishes – a paternalistic act. As the client passes through the acute phase of illness towards recovery, it may be that he or she subsequently ratifies the paternalistic actions of the health care team. Perhaps the client may point out that looking back on the incident of being given medication against their wishes, they now recognise they were ill at that time and are now pleased that the team did not respect their utterances but instead gave the medication. For another example, consider that a very young child refuses to go to the dentist in spite of his parents' exhortations (adapted from Benjamin and Curtis, 1986, p. 53). Eventually, the parents coerce the child into visiting the dentist. The child, having now grown up with beautiful teeth, recalls the struggles with his parents which visits to the dentist caused. Recognising that his parents were, after all, acting in his best interests, he informs them that he is now pleased they acted against his wishes and coerced him into undergoing dental treatment. In such an example, the child ratifies the paternalistic actions of his parents.

One may feel justifiably suspicious with respect to the ratification condition. It seems to require that health care professionals peer into the future to speculate upon the client's attitude at a later time to the paternalistic intervention. If health care professionals do not know a client well, it seems likely that the ratification condition could be open to abuse. This must constitute a grave concern as far as the adoption and application of this condition is concerned.

Having expressed that, quite serious, reservation it does seem that there are circumstances under which the ratification condition is a legitimate posit, and in which the possibility of its abuse may be minimised. For example, in the context of mental health nursing, it is often the case that nurses build up relationships with clients (and their relatives) which are quite long-standing. A nurse may well feel with good reason that they are in a good position to make a judgement about what the client would want to happen in a particular type of situation. Perhaps, over time, the nurse has come to learn of the client's attitudes and values. It may even be supposed that certain possible future events have been discussed between the nurse and the client. For example, suppose a client is said to suffer from schizophrenia. The client undergoes a recognisable cycle of acute breakdown, and medication-sustained recovery. It may be that the nurse could determine during the client's stable, illness-free periods just what kinds of intervention they would prefer to happen in the event of the onset of an acute phase of the illness. It may be, for example, that the nurse could put to the client the question: 'In the event of you refusing to take medication at some point in the future (within specified limits), would you prefer your wishes expressed at that future time to be respected, or your wishes now to be respected?' In a situation such as that, it seems, the notion of retrospective ratification does have some reasonable application. Perhaps so-called 'Community Supervision Orders' could be organised along these lines (see, for example, Bluglass, 1993).

Thus far then, we have considered Benjamin and Curtis's criteria for determining whether or not a paternalistic intervention is justified. In their position, as we saw, all three conditions need to be met before such an intervention is justified. That is to say, a person must meet the following three criteria:

- The client must not be competent at the relevant time (the person must meet the autonomy condition);
- It must be the case that the course of action pursued by the client is highly likely to result in significant harm to the client (the person must meet the harm condition);
- It must be the case that the client is highly likely to ratify the proposed paternalistic intervention at some later time (the person must meet the ratification condition).

It should be said that given our comments on the notion of competence in Chapter 3 previously, the first condition is perhaps better described as a 'competence condition', since the relevant question concerns the competence of the client, but perhaps this minor point can be passed over. The second condition has been commented on. With respect to the third, the reservations expressed above concerning its application seem serious; but, as indicated above, in cases where there is a therapeutic relationship of sufficient depth which obtains between the nurse and the client, then a role can be envisaged for the ratification condition. But, in other cases, for example where the wishes of the client are not known and there are no friends or relatives of the client to indicate the client's beliefs and values, then it is hard to envisage a defensible role for the ratification condition. Hence, it does not seem plausible to include satisfaction of the ratification condition in a list of necessary or sufficient conditions relevant to the justification of paternalistic interventions. More plausibly, in certain types of case, a ratification condition may comprise a necessary but not a sufficient condition of justified paternalism.

Given these comments, then, the following conclusion can be advanced. Paternalistic interventions are only justified when the client is not competent. This conclusion is entirely congenial to the general position being tentatively advanced in this work: it is one in which the principle of respect for autonomy is being accorded the greatest of moral weight (due to the considerations advanced in Chapter 3 and in the above discussion of paternalism).

Suicidal clients

It needs to be said that the position arrived at here implies that it is not possible to justify preventing a person from committing suicide who has made a competent decision to do so. In fact, in the position tentatively endorsed here it is not possible justifiably to prevent any competent person from harming themselves. Rightly, theorists from other theoretical perspectives express concern about such a position (as should all proponents of an autonomy-weighted, principle-based approach). It seems excessively harsh and uncaring to state baldly that a competent person should not be prevented from committing suicide. Hence, it is necessary to offer some views on this extremely difficult and distressing issue.

Rational decisions to commit suicide

A first position to be set aside here is the view that anyone who decides to end their own life must be sufficiently mentally unwell that they cannot competently make such a decision, and, hence, that paternalistic interventions are justified in such cases. (Glover, 1977, p. 171, suggests that such a view is held by certain theorists.) In response to such a position, it is worth considering a case example offered by Bloch and Heyd (1981, p. 198). They describe the case of a 65-year-old man who has cancer of the colon with 'widespread secondaries'. He has only a few weeks left to live and states:

> [He] would rather die 'with dignity' and in full possession of his senses than in excruciating pain which calls for massive doses of narcotic drugs.

The man seeks to acquire a 'sufficient number of hypnotic pills' in order to end his own life – in the way in which he wants it to end. (See also *The Last Right: the need for voluntary euthanasia,* Voluntary Euthanasia Society, 1992.)

The clear implication of Bloch and Heyd's discussion is that it is indeed perfectly rational for the person they describe to decide to commit suicide. His remaining few weeks of life promise only continued suffering and inevitable death. It seems entirely rational, given such terrible prospects, to desire to avoid that avoidable and pointless period of suffering. The publication referred to in the last note contains descriptions of similar, equally distressing case examples.

Given acceptance of the claim that there can be suicidal acts which are rational – that result from competent decisions to do so – it needs to be made explicit that it does not thereby follow that all suicidal acts are rational. It is evident that a person's suicidal feelings may well result from a transient mood or mental health problem. Indeed, certain kinds of mental health problems are particularly associated with the risk of suicide (for example, depression, schizophrenia and alcoholism).

It may be useful to draw attention to a continuum of types of cases. At one end we find those in which an autonomous person makes a competent decision to end their own life. Perhaps the example provided by Bloch and Heyd above constitutes such a case. At the other end are to be found cases in which the person is not autonomous and is clearly not competent to decide to take his or her own life. Perhaps a person is in the acute phase of schizophrenia and wishes to end her life due to the perceived presence of a venomous snake in her stomach. In between these two poles of the continuum there are a variety of much more difficult types of cases in which it is not clear to what degree the person is competent to make a decision to commit suicide.

Given what was said earlier concerning paternalistic interventions, it should be clear that justifying such interventions is much less problematic in the cases where the client is not competent and, also, even where the client's competence is in doubt.

In cases of the kind described by Bloch and Heyd above, it is relatively easy to appreciate that the decision made by the client is a rational one, when the future promises only certain death and pain. It is plausible that paternalistic interventions designed to prevent such a person from committing suicide are extremely hard to justify. Certainly, employing the schema of Benjamin and Curtis (1986), such a person would seem to meet none of their conditions necessary to justify paternalistic interventions. The person fails to satisfy the autonomy condition; the person will come to significant harm whether prevented or 'permitted' to end their own life; and it is extremely unlikely, given the client's reasons for committing suicide, that they would later ratify actions designed to prevent them taking their own life.

Much more difficult cases are those in which a person wishes to end their own life on the grounds that the future appears to promise a greater amount of suffering than of pleasure, and so decides to end life now rather than endure the anticipated suffering. Such a person decides that life is simply not worth living.

It is not hard to envisage circumstances in which a person might well consider suicide on the basis of the likelihood that life has little to offer. Indeed, Camus claims that 'All healthy men [and women?] have thought of their own suicide' (1955, p. 13). It certainly seems to be the case that persons other than those suffering from a terminal illness, or extremely debilitating health problem, seriously consider suicide. Given this, an autonomy-weighted position implies that it is not justifiable to prevent such a person from taking their own life. This

conclusion seems sufficiently jarring to warrant further attention: it seems that emotional factors seek to override logical
conclusions here. This is, indeed, a commonly voiced criticism
of the principle-based approach, and one which will be returned to in Chapter 5.

In his discussion of suicide, Harris (1985) seems adamant that
persons who make competent decisions to end their own lives
cannot justifiably be prevented from doing so (Harris, 1985,
p. 203; also Beauchamp and Childress, 1989, p. 226). But
Glover in his discussion (1977, ch. 13) and Bloch and Heyd
(1981) are less sure. For example, Bloch and Heyd point to a
special, perhaps unique, feature of suicidal acts, namely their
irreversibility (1981, p. 200). They identify an asymmetry between decisions not to prevent a suicidal act, and decisions to
prevent such an act. Obviously, if a suicidal act is successfully
undertaken, there are no opportunities available for the suicidal person to reconsider his views. But, if a person is prevented
from committing suicide, then such an opportunity is made
available. This asymmetry may be taken to warrant a stance in
which it is justifiable to prevent a person committing suicide –
at least to give the person more time to consider his views. In
fact, Glover suggests that it is 'always legitimate' (1977, p. 176)
to reason with a person who expresses suicidal intentions.
He claims that such an intervention does not amount to a
violation of respect for autonomy. Further, perhaps surpris-
ingly, he claims that it is legitimate to 'restrain by force' (1977,
p. 177) a person who is not persuaded against suicide by rational means. The view seems to be that if a person is sufficiently determined to take his own life, then he can simply do so at
a future date.

So, the paternalistic stance apparently endorsed by Glover
and by Bloch and Heyd, stems from the claim that due to the
special nature of suicidal actions – the asymmetry between
intervention and non-intervention – the general obligations to
respect autonomy can be overridden.

This position clearly deserves sympathy, but there may be
some difficulty in sustaining the claimed asymmetry between
decisions to intervene to prevent suicide, and decisions not to
intervene. Other examples of irreversible actions may include
giving away all one's property, and possibly other types of acts,

but, clearly these would not be of the same gravity as suicidal acts.

However, placing such a heavy weight upon irreversibility may not, in the end, be plausible. This is due to the possibility that a proponent of an autonomy-weighted position may counter by arguing in two ways. First, such a theorist might point out that the appeal to irreversibility is simply a red herring. The moral dilemma raised by suicidal intentions stems from a conflict between respect for autonomy and other moral principles (nonmaleficence for example); this is the real issue, such a theorist may say. Hence, the irreversibility or otherwise of suicidal acts is wholly irrelevant to the issue of justifiable interventions to prevent suicide. Second, such a theorist might go further and put forward the view that the very fact that suicidal acts are irreversible, renders them of such significance that they should simply be left to the actor. So, it seems not to be the case that much mileage can be gleaned from Bloch and Heyd's suggestion – at least as far as the present author can discern; and, hence, that paternalistic interventions are no easier to justify in relations to suicidal clients than in clients whose actions present other types of moral problems. Given this rather uncomfortable conclusion, let us now move on to consider conflicts between respect for autonomy and the principle of justice.

Autonomy in conflict with justice: allocation of scarce resources

Four criteria may be considered concerning the fair allocation of health care resources. These are that health care resources should be allocated: according to need; according to desert; according to right; and according to utility – which may be referred to, respectively, as needs-based, desert-based, rights-based, and utility-based criteria. Roughly, these are the criteria which Gillon claims were suggested by his eight-year-old daughter (Gillon, 1985, p. 95; also Beauchamp and Childress, 1989, p. 261).

Before moving on to consider these four criteria, other points of clarification are required. First, how is the term 'allocation' to be understood in questions concerning resource allocation? It is customary to draw a distinction between macroallocation, mesoallocation, and microallocation of health care resources (see, for example, Gillon, 1985, ch. 15; Beauchamp and Childress, 1989, ch. 6). Rather crudely, questions of macroallocation concern the proportion of the finances available to a government which is to be allocated to health care – as opposed to, say, arms and education. Microallocation of resources is said by Gillon to involve decisions such as choosing between 'competing claimants' (1985, p. 93) for, say, a kidney dialysis machine or a place in a special care baby unit. And mesoallocation concerns questions of distribution of resources between the macro and micro-levels (say at regional level, or at hospital level).

From the specifically nursing perspective, it can be pointed out that nurses regularly make decisions concerning the way they should divide the time they spend with clients. Of course, nursing time is itself a health care resource (Dickenson, 1994). For example, a community nurse with a large case-load may have to decide which is the fairest way to manage that case-load. Inevitably less time will be allocated to certain clients than to others. But which criteria will the nurse invoke in order to make such a decision? Similarly, in a ward situation, a nurse may be aware that there is only a limited supply of bed linen available for the clients she is directly responsible for. How should she decide which clients will receive clean linen, and which ones will have to make do? So, nurses evidently have to make decisions at the level of microallocation, and probably at the level of mesoallocation also. But, further, the UKCC Code (UKCC, 1992, clause 11) appears to require that nurses concern themselves with the values which inform macroallocation of health care resources. This issue is returned to at the end of the present section.

By way of further clarification, it should be noted that health care ranges from care given in the hospital setting, to care given in the community, in addition to health education and promotion. And resources should be taken to include personnel (medical, nursing, administrative, ancillary, and so on), equipment, research findings, research projects, and buildings necessary for the implementation of health care.

Utility-based criteria (specifically, social utility)

Applied to Gillon's example of a case involving competing claimants for a kidney dialysis machine, a utility-based criterion would determine that the machine should go to the person whose continued survival would generate the greatest amount of (social) utility. For example, one commentator, Rescher, proposes:

> [In] its allocation [of health care resources] society 'invests' a scarce resource in one person as against another and is thus entitled to look to the probable prospective 'return' on its investment.
> (N. Rescher, quoted in Beauchamp and Childress, 1989, p. 299)

Presumably, the 'returns' referred to here are to be understood in material terms. For example, in terms of how much a person can contribute to the economic development of the relevant society, or whether he or she has children whose potential to contribute to the particular society would be enhanced by the continued survival of the client. It seems plausible that allocation of health care resources along these lines would inevitably favour younger people at the expense of older people, since it seems more likely that the former will have dependants, and that they will be employed – especially given an upper age limit on eligibility for employment, as in the UK.

As might be anticipated, utility-based criteria can be subjected to a number of criticisms. First, as noted above, it seems that the criterion contains an inbuilt bias towards the young and the economically productive. Apart from objections on other grounds, it may be the case that the citizens of such a society come to recognise that they are only valued when they are economically productive, or young. In the light of this, they may decide to go and live elsewhere in a society which has other values. So it is possible that application of the (social) utility-based criterion may turn out to result in a longer-term disutility.

Second, a query arises relating to the consistency of the utility-based view. Recall the quote from Rescher offered earlier. Might not an older person who has contributed taxes to the state during a lengthy working life claim that *they* are entitled to a 'return' on their investment?

Third, it would seem to follow from the adoption of a social utility criterion that, say, a 35-year-old person who arrives in a particular country never having previously visited there, nor contributed anything to the country by payment of taxes, would have a greater chance of receiving scarce resources than a person who has paid taxes for 50 years and is now aged 80. This offends intuitive views of justice as 'desert' (cf. Chapter 3 above).

Fourth, cases in which there is a clear contrast between the respective utility of two candidates for resources can mask difficulties in the utility-based view. Such difficulties can be exposed by consideration of other types of case. For example, suppose a 25-year-old person and a 26-year-old person are competing for scarce resources; also that they are each in need of similar care, and have similar qualifications, skills and so forth. It seems simply arbitrary from the moral perspective to claim that the resource should go to the younger person on the grounds that that person has more opportunities (one extra year) to contribute to the economy of the relevant society. Such a position seems open to many of the standard difficulties which dog Utilitarianism; these include difficulties in predicting consequences of actions, or policies of resource allocation.

A rights-based criterion

Given the apparent obstacles to acceptance of a utility-based criterion, perhaps a rights-based criterion may prove viable. According to this view, health care resources go to those who have a right to them. The plausibility of this view stems in part from the increasingly widespread employment of appeals to rights. One hears of the rights of the unborn child, the rights of women over their own bodies, rights to health care, to privacy, to education, to free speech, to silence, to information and so on. And, of course, *The Patient's Charter* (Department of Health, 1991) seems to constitute an example of an attempt to anchor claims relating to provision of health care resources in the language of rights.

It is important to draw attention to two distinct types of rights; those which make demands upon material resources and those which do not. Rights of the first kind include rights to education; health care for example. Clearly, in order for it to be possible for these rights to be met, certain material conditions have to be in place. For rights to health care to be met, it follows that the resources necessary to provide that care need to be in place; similarly, with rights to education, shelter, and food. A different type of rights does not seem so obviously dependent upon the availability of material resources – perhaps the right to free speech is one such.

Rights of the first kind are described by Beauchamp and Childress as 'positive rights' (1989, p. 59): these invoke the 'right to be provided with a particular good or service by others'. Hence, rights to health care resources are describable as positive rights; for example, the right to receive certain benefits.

Let us now consider some difficulties in employing a rights-based criterion. First, in cases of the kind referred to by Gillon (1985) – namely, those which involve equally legitimate claims on limited resources (kidney machines, special-care baby unit places) – the appeal to rights seems entirely otiose. If only one machine or bed is available, the unlucky person may appeal to her right to receive the treatment, but it does not follow from this that she will receive it.

It may be countered that in the health care context, all one has a right to is a decent minimum level of health care (Beauchamp and Childress, 1989, p. 275). But there are obvious difficulties with such a proposal. A decent minimum may reasonably be taken to include heart transplants, IVF and the provision of expensive drugs.

Second, it is common to point out that the language of rights is only intelligible given acceptance of 'the correlativity thesis' (Beauchamp and Childress, 1989, p. 57; Frey, 1983). The claim here is that in the case of positive rights, such rights are only meaningful given the availability of the material resources available to meet them. But in cases where equally needy clients demand scarce resources, appeals to rights seem to fail to meet the correlativity thesis. Further, given such situations, it seems inevitable that other criteria for allocating resources will be invoked – perhaps, Utilitarian criteria – or that the resource will be allocated on an entirely *ad hoc* basis.

A needs-based criterion

According to this criterion, resources should go to those who need them. On the face of it, this seems an intuitively plausible answer. If a person needs a health care resource, then they should be given it. In fact, *The Patient's Charter* (Department of Health, 1991, p. 8) seems to state a commitment to a needs-based criterion. According to it, 'Every citizen has the [right] to receive health care on the basis of clinical need, regardless of ability to pay' (see also Daniels, 1985).

But, of course, there are a number of serious difficulties with such a view. An initial difficulty arises since, clearly, no geographical boundaries are set in the criterion as it stands. To claim simply that resources should go to those who need them, involves setting no criteria for the determination of eligibility to the resources other than 'clinical need'. But, typically, it will be asserted that national boundaries affect one's entitlement to the relevant resources and, hence, that priority will be given to members of a particular society. So, the needs-based criterion, more properly, should be taken to claim that: within a specified parameter X, resources should go to those who need them (where 'X' stands for a national boundary).

A further difficulty for the needs-based view stems from problems distinguishing needs from mere wants. For example, Seedhouse proposes that in matters of health care provision, 'basic needs [should be met] before any other want' (1988, p. 132). For this claim to mean much we need, at least, a definition of the term 'need'. Beauchamp and Childress write:

> [To] say that a person needs something is to say that without it the person will be harmed (or at least detrimentally affected). (1989, p. 260)

This may be a little too weak, however. Presumably, needs include any life-threatening condition. It is easy to appreciate that medical conditions such as heart trouble, peritonitis, and pneumonia place their sufferers in need of medical treatment. One might attempt to contrast those in need of treatments for such conditions with those who merely want some kind of medical intervention – say, counselling, psychotherapy or cosmetic surgery. But this intuitive division comes under threat since, it seems, any want can be transformed into a need. This follows since a person may claim to be suicidal if denied access to interventions of the kind just referred to. Hence, in this way, a needs-based criterion can seem too weak since it could include interventions usually regarded as mere wants.

In a different way, a needs-based criterion could seem too strong. This is due to the temptation to take a strong line and argue that anything one can live without is a mere want and is not a need. Thus, needs would cover only life-threatening conditions. To see that this is too strong, one need only consider interventions such as eye operations which restore an individual's sight (say, cataract removal), and hip replacements. Each of these types of interventions bestow high opportunities for quality of life improvement on their recipients; also, they are relatively inexpensive procedures. So, it would be implausible to exclude interventions such as these on the basis of the fact that they are not life-threatening.

Further, a needs-based view is vulnerable to one of the same objections which besets a rights-based view; namely, how to cope with situations in which equally needy clients require a scarce resource. Evidently, the needs-based criterion is as redundant here as is the rights-based criterion.

So, a commitment to meeting health care needs from a needs-based perspective seems open to at least three substantial objections. There is a problem in specifying just who is potentially entitled to the relevant resources: is it restricted to residents of a specific country or not? Then there is the apparent difficulty that any want can be transformed into a need. Also, there is a temptation to try to ground a distinction between wants and needs by appeal to the life-threatening nature, or otherwise, of specific medical conditions. But this can make the needs-based line far too strong, in that it excludes interventions such as cataract operations and hip replacements.

A desert-based criterion

Obviously enough, according to this criterion, health care resources go to those who deserve them. In Gillon's example, the machine would go to the person who had done most to deserve it. This proposal raises the question of what kinds of activities a person needs to perform in order to be said to deserve health care resources? Here are some suggestions.

- One (implausible) answer may be that a person must have performed certain types of positive actions – actions which have benefited one's country. These may include fighting for one's country, developing a cure for a serious illness, or, say, working in the nursing or medical professions.
- A less demanding construal of desert may require merely that the person concerned has contributed financially to the nation's health budget by way of payment of taxes.
- A still less demanding construal would be one in which desert is construed negatively, so to speak. Hence, rather than require that individuals have performed certain types of act, it may be said that persons are entitled to health care resources providing they have abstained from specified types of actions. For example, it may be proposed that one is entitled to health care resources providing one has not done anything to render one undeserving of these resources. Examples of actions which may render one undeserving may include performing highly antisocial actions such as murder; or merely that one knowingly exposed oneself unnecessarily to risks of ill-health (perhaps by smoking, heavy drinking, or not exercising (?)). Persons who engage in such courses of action may be said to forfeit their desert to health care resources.

It is worth pointing out that adoption of a desert-based criterion may be thought to favour older people at the expense of younger people. This may be the case since the longer a person lives, the greater the opportunities they have had to perform actions such as those referred to in the first two items above. Hence, a desert-based view may redress some of the imbalance which appears to be present in utility-based views, for example.

With respect to the notion of 'negative desert' referred to in the third item above, this could be recruited to ensure that the very young would still have a legitimate claim to health care resources. The specification here also carries the possible merit that those unable to make an economic contribution to a particular society would still be entitled to health care resources – providing they refrained from actions which render them un- deserving. Let us turn, now, to consider some of the difficulties raised by proposal of a desert-based criterion.

A first possible difficulty with the desert-based view is that it appears to be an extremely harsh policy. To focus on the two positive types of criteria referred to above would seem to ex- clude large numbers of the population, and this simply is not acceptable. The inclusion of considerations relating to negative desert may also appear excessively harsh. It may be that a person damages their liver by years of heavy drinking. Should such a person be denied access to treatment for the liver dam- age on the grounds that they brought it upon themselves? Intuitions vary here, but it seems very harsh to judge that the person has forfeited their claim to health care resources. Aside from these points, John Harris (BBC TV, 'Heart of the matter: rationing health care', 27/6/93) has raised what seems an ex- tremely difficult problem for the position when it involves appeals to negative desert. The criticism Harris raises is that the fair operation of such a system would require, in effect, the appointment of a 'lifestyle police'. The activities of each citizen would need close and careful monitoring to ensure that each unhealthy action or behaviour is recorded, so that it can be deployed against the citizen should they require health care resources at some future time. Harris thus regards the level of intrusiveness apparently required for the fair implementation of a desert-based view as wholly unacceptable. This seems to constitute a serious, if not fatal, blow to this view: without the inclusion of negative desert it excludes too many citizens; but when negative desert is included, consideration of the practicalities of applying the criterion weigh heavily against its adoption.

Finally, there are two other worries concerning the desert- based view. First, it is not clear how the criterion would apply to new arrivals in a society – be they neonates or people from other countries wishing to settle in that society. If shortly after arrival they require health care resources, how should this situation be coped with? Again, to deny access to resources sounds brutally harsh. Second, the desert-based view appears to face the same difficulty faced by the other three criteria that have been considered: specifically, how to cope with situations in which equally deserving cases are competing for scarce resources and where both claims cannot be met.

Combining criteria?

Given that each of the four positions considered seems equally problematic, it may be proposed that the criteria be combined in some way. Such a proposal might recommend that, as a general rule, resources should go to those who need them; but, where this is not possible, other sorts of considerations should be taken into account. So, needing a health care resource marks one as a possible candidate for the receipt of resources, and then other criteria may be brought in to play in the assessment of one's claim. For example, the notions of desert or utility may be said to buttress a claim for resources equally strongly. This approach may help to avoid criticism of the utility-based view to the effect that it unfairly discriminates against older people; and, it may temper the possible bias towards older people in the desert-based view. In spite of difficulties other than that just mentioned which beset the desert-based position, it may well be the case that the last proposal has some merit. This may be due to the fact that, as we saw in Chapter 3 earlier, desert does seem to comprise a significant component of our understanding of the concept of justice. More controversially, the same may be claimed of the notion of utility. So, perhaps a feasible criterion of fair distribution can be derived by combining need, utility and desert in some way.

However, a more profitable way forward may be to reconsider relevant moral principles here. In the earlier discussion of justice, Rawls's theory was considered; and it will be recalled that this may be described as a contractarian view. Given the apparent plausibility of the claim that great weight should be accorded to obligations to respect autonomy, it may be suggested that the whole question of how best to allocate resources should be resolved by appeal to what may be termed 'collective autonomy': such decisions should be left to those potentially affected by them. Such a suggestion, in fact, seems to be one for which Rawls's hypothetical 'original position' could be invoked, as discussed in the previous chapter. For example, it may be put to the subjects in the original position that some access to health care provision should be built in to the state, since it is of course possible that any one of them could be poor and fall ill, or have a condition which requires medical resources (say, diabetes). (For development of such a view, see Green, 1976; and Daniels, 1985.)

Also, such a proposal seems to have the merit of being founded upon respect for the autonomous decisions of subjects and, thereby on the principle of respect for autonomy. Subjects are being given the opportunity to make informed decisions (decisions based upon awareness of the costs and outcomes of various treatment options) concerning how best to allocate limited resources. It should be emphasised that such a proposal changes the emphasis of questions relating to the distribution of resources. The change is from a consideration of who should be treated, to consideration of which conditions should be treated (Sipes-Metzler, 1994).

Given acceptance of earlier arguments reporting the importance of autonomy in nursing ethics, it follows that basing a policy of allocation of resources on the principle of respect for autonomy seems well-founded from the moral perspective. Such a proposal has been attempted in practice in Oregon, USA (Sipes-Metzler, 1994; Capuzzi and Garland, 1990; and Barker, 1995). Should its acceptance be recommended in the UK? Although such a proposal may seem plausible from the moral perspective, there are some serious problems with it, and whether these problems are insurmountable or not I will leave for the reader to judge.

First, in the Oregon Plan, types of health care interventions were prioritised in accordance with 'public values and medical facts' (Sipes-Metzler, 1994, p. 305; see also Capuzzi and Garland, 1990, p. 261). These were obtained from a series of public meetings and telephone surveys. However, grounding public policy on public values may lead to objectionable consequences. For example, given that ageism is widespread in Western cultures, it is not unlikely that programmes of allocation of resources which benefit younger citizens at the expense of older ones would be considered acceptable. Further, there are the kinds of health care problems which are associated – justly or unjustly – with lifestyles or ethnic groups disapproved of by many citizens; AIDS and drug dependence spring to mind here. In short, the worry is that irrational prejudices which are widespread among citizens may work themselves into policy concerning distribution of resources.

Second, in contrast to the last worry, it may turn out to be the case that the reports of public values obtained from public meetings and so forth, fail to give an accurate representation of the values held by the majority of citizens. This may be due to the fact that only politically active citizens attend the meetings; or citizens who, say, are employed in health-related occupations (see Benjamin and Curtis, 1992, p. 202).

Third, it is evident that the public perception of sufferers from certain medical conditions differs from that of sufferers from other types of medical conditions. For example, people with illnesses such as AIDS may be regarded as in some way to blame for their health problems; especially if that condition is associated with lifestyles which many members of the population disapprove of (for example, those involving intravenous drug use and sexual relations between members of the same sex). These types of prejudices are highly likely to emerge in surveys which poll the attitudes of citizens to certain ways of prioritising distribution of health care resources; and this may be morally offensive.

Fourth, it may be suggested that the public should not be consulted since they are not experts on health care matters. Hence, this objection queries the legitimacy of the whole approach taken in Oregon and which appears to follow from the emphasis placed on autonomy in the present volume.

Fifth, it may be said that the system of distribution put forward in the Oregon plan is unfair to poor people. This is because rich people will always be able to meet their health needs by purchasing from the private sector. Hence, only poorer citizens will be detrimentally affected by the implementation of the plan.

Responses

When one considers these objections a pattern emerges. The first objection points to a problem in ensuring that the process of consulting the citizens is democratic, in that not all those entitled to express a view may do so; similarly with the second objection. The third and fourth objections ˙tacitly refer to ancient problems with any democratic system. Specifically, these suggest that since members of the electorate are not experts, then they are not qualified to make judgements – concerning, for example, matters of government or, for that matter, allocation of health care resources.

These objections to democracy were set out persuasively by Plato (see *The Republic*). We may describe them as objections concerning the inadequacy of democracy. However, the fact is that the political systems in place in Western cultures are all (at least supposedly) democratic; the selection of governments is performed by the electorate at election times. Surely, if this system of selection of governments is considered acceptable, then it should be considered acceptable when applied to the question of how to distribute health care resources.

The suggestion here, then, is that objections stemming from the claimed inadequacy of the democratic process, or from democracy itself as a political system, are not sufficient to count against the kind of proposal put forward in the Oregon Plan. For, if governments are best chosen by vote, surely systems for the distribution of health care resources are also.

The fifth objection stated that a system of distribution along the lines of the Oregon Plan is unfair to economically disadvantaged people. This is due to the fact that they alone will bear any harms which result from rationing of resources (at least within the relevant population group). The reason why this charge is legitimate can be seen by reconsideration of points made in our discussion of justice.

Suppose two citizens are each covered by a nationwide health plan in which the system of distribution of health care resources is based upon the autonomous wishes of the electorate – call it the UK-Plan. Suppose further that each of our two citizens are in need of an expensive health care intervention which is unlikely to be forthcoming in the terms of the UK-Plan. Such an intervention may be a highly expensive transplant operation, or 24-hour nursing care in the client's own home.

Let us judge that each of these two clients is equally needy; however, let us suppose that one client is very rich and can afford to pay for the expensive health care intervention, but the other client is poor and cannot afford to pay. According to our earlier formulation of the principle of justice in Chapter 3, we are to treat equals equally. If the relevant respect in which these two clients are equals is that they are equally needy of a specific health care resource, then the poorer client can claim to be the victim of an injustice. For, equals have not been treated equally and, hence, the principle of justice has been violated.

It is important to tread carefully here. As seen earlier, for Rawls, certain properties of individuals are not morally relevant. If it is supposed that the rich client became rich fortuitously – say by virtue of a large inheritance – it may be argued that the two clients are indeed equals from the moral perspective. But a morally relevant difference may be claimed to obtain between the rich client and the poor one. For example, this may be said to be the case if the rich client obtained his riches from years of lengthy and hard labour combined with skilful and risky financial judgements.

It is not necessary to comment further here on ways of defending the view that the poorer client is the victim of an injustice, or not. Suffice to say that if one favours Nozick's theory of justice described in the previous chapter, one will be more likely to judge that the poorer client is not the victim of an injustice – merely the victim of misfortune. If one favours a Rawlsian criterion, then one may be much more sympathetic to the claim that the poorer client is indeed dealt an unjust blow.

The discussion so far has not focused on matters of allocation at the micro-level – at the level of nursing practice. But it is clear that nurses do require an understanding of possible approaches to questions of resource allocation (as noted earlier, perhaps the UKCC Code even obliges nurses to have such an understanding).

At the micro-level, nurses, their time and their skills all constitute health care resources. So, a decision taken by a nurse regarding how to manage their time whilst on duty, is a decision concerning resource allocation. As noted, the UKCC Code provides a framework of constraints within which nurses have to make decisions. It is not an option to allocate one's time and skills in such a way that one client is benefited greatly but another is negligently ignored. To plan a regime of care in such a way would be a clear breach of the UKCC Code. Hence, nurses' decisions regarding how to allocate their time and skills are constrained by their professional obligations. Given this, a CPN, say, with a given case-load is obliged to manage his or her time so that the well-being of all clients can be met. This seems to indicate that the criteria for just allocation of nursing time and skills are needs-based: nurses are obliged to try to meet the health care needs of those in their care. This applies to nurses in all contexts. Difficulties arise when nurses find themselves unable to meet such needs, and where this is due to factors beyond their control. For example, it may be the case that in order to meet the needs of clients, more nurses or more equipment are required. It becomes evident at this point that matters of microallocation are related, eventually, to matters of macroallocation; since, if it is not possible for nurses to meet the needs of their clients given existing resources, decisions have to be made at macro-level concerning questions of health care priorities. Decisions at that level can be influenced by the nurse as a health care professional and as a citizen.

Situations in which nurses are unable to meet the needs of their clients in the sense required by the UKCC Code, and in which further resources are not forthcoming, will receive attention in Chapter 6 below.

This chapter began by discussing moral dilemmas which arise from conflicts between the principles of respect for autonomy, and those of beneficence and nonmaleficence. This led into a discussion of the conditions under which paternalistic interventions may be justified, and a discussion of clients who wish to kill or harm themselves. It was, reluctantly, concluded that an autonomy-weighted, principle-based line appears to imply that paternalistic interventions in such instances are extremely hard to justify. An important exemplification of conflict between obligations generated by respect for autonomy, and those generated by the principle of justice was then considered; specifically in relation to the allocation of health care resources. After consideration of a number of criteria (utility, rights and so on) a tentative proposal founded on respect for 'collective autonomy' was advanced.

5 A challenge to the principle-based approach

The present chapter discusses a challenge to the principle-based approach from a rival theoretical standpoint – that of a care-based approach to ethics. Since the chapter will involve, in effect, a debate between these two positions, it may be useful to clarify in advance of the discussion certain key issues.

As seen, crudely, the principle-based approach to nursing ethics endorses the adoption of a general strategy. The strategy involves application of four moral principles to moral problems encountered by nurses. Arguments were offered earlier, in Chapter 3, in support of the claim that the obligations generated by the principle of respect for autonomy are the most weighty of the obligations generated by the four principles we have considered.

With regard to the care-based approach this can be problematic to summarise, but four general commitments can be identified. First, it is argued that moral problems are unique (call this *The Uniqueness Claim*); and, hence, that general approaches to moral problems such as that represented by the principle-based approach, are fundamentally misconceived. Moral problems are thought unique since no two people are exactly the same and no two people will be involved in exactly the same set of relations with others. Second, it is pointed out that persons are typically involved in caring relationships with significant others (family and, in the case of nurses, clients). Moral problems arise in the context of such relationships (call this *The Caring Claim*). Third, it is held that the experiencing of such problems is accompanied by the experiencing of emotions and feelings (call this *The Emotions Claim*). And, fourth, it is suggested that those involved in the relevant problem will have a view of it which differs from, and is more relevant to the problem than, views held by those outside the particular 'web' of relationships (call this *The Privileged View Claim*). This, in a nutshell, is a very crude outline of the care-based view.

It should be clear how these key aspects of the care-based approach conflict with a crude version of the principle-based view. First, the alleged uniqueness of moral problems – The Uniqueness Claim – seems to be denied in the principle-based view, in which a great number of moral problems can be analysed in the same way (by determining which principles clash). Second, the principle-based view seems silent on the issue of caring relations – on The Caring Claim (as will be seen, shortly, this leads to the charge of callousness). Third, the principle-based view is silent on the relation between emotions and moral thinking – The Emotions Claim. And, fourth, the principle-based view seems to accord no special insight into moral problems to those involved in them – The Privileged View Claim.

The care-based view will be discussed in more detail in the remainder of this chapter, but, for the moment, it is hoped that the reader now has an indication of the main differences between the care-based and principle-based approaches.

The discussion begins with certain concerns about the principle-based approach. This is followed by an attempt to characterise the care-based view, and a number of problems associated with it are identified. It is argued that care is not the essence of nursing, and a defence of the principle-based view is attempted. Finally, a position is put forward which remains recognisably principle-based, but which takes on certain of the legitimate worries which proponents of a care-based approach have with regard to the principle-based line.

Concerns about the principle-based approach

Too callous and uncaring

The discussion in the previous chapter of the moral problems surrounding persons who express suicidal intentions, brought to the fore a certain type of worry which commentators have about the principle-based approach to ethics. It can seem excessively harsh and unfeeling simply to judge that if a person makes a competent, autonomous decision to end their life, then this should be respected. Further, this conclusion is one which seems to follow from arguments relating to the various weightings attached to the principles. Given a position motivated by such arguments, logic can draw us to certain conclusions which our emotions incline us to reject. Alderson, for example, draws attention to the suggestion that approaches to ethics which emphasise respect for autonomy, have '. . . a chilly, uncaring emphasis on respect as non-interference' (1992, p. 33).

The general charge, here, seems to be that application of the principle-based approach in practice conflicts to such an extent with the moral intuitions and emotions of practitioners, that the approach should be abandoned. A possible example of similar worries being expressed in relation to moral reasoning arises in an exchange between John Harris and Mark Hockey. They are discussing the hypothetical example of two clients, one aged 70 and one aged 30, who are both in need of the single available bed in an intensive care unit.

> [Harris]:   On the assumption that both of [the clients] are equally entitled to the care of the community, we shouldn't choose between them, and therefore we should toss a coin as to who gets the bed.
> [Hockey]:   I think Professor Harris's comments were quite valid in terms of a concept of pure ethics, but we do not live in a world of pure ethics. We live in a world of having to make practical decisions . . . on the ground, his advice would be of little practical help . . . (BBC, 1994, p. 31; see also Harris, 1985, p. 40)

In this exchange, we seem to have the clash between emotional and logical considerations which implementation of the principle-based approach can invoke, and which leads certain theorists to reject it.

Too simplistic

The charge that the principle-based view is overly simplistic is also a criticism raised by certain commentators. The suggestion seems to be that moral problems are much too complicated to be viewed through the lens of the principle-based approach. The approach leaves out too much that is central to the nature of moral problems; for example, the emotional elements experienced by persons involved in the relevant moral problem. As Alderson puts it, 'Some bio-ethicists try to reduce morality to two or three principles, then decide which should be the winning principle if they clash' (1992, p. 33). Her clear implication here, is that this is far too simplistic and wholly inappropriate. As with Alderson, Hunt expresses concerns that adoption of the principle-based approach can make it seem that moral problems are as easy to solve as problems in arithmetic (Hunt, 1994a, p. 5).

Too complicated and jargon-laden (Hunt, 1994a, p. 4)

Hunt's other concerns appear to be that adoption and implementation of a principle-based approach to nursing ethics is merely an attempt to render ethics more scientific or medical. Crudely, the suggestion seems to be that it is presumed in health care, in general, that technology and specialisation are desirable, good things. Hunt is justly wary, and perhaps even hostile to such a view. The introduction of the principle-based approach in nursing curricula is simply another symptom of this general malaise.

Hunt points out that students enter into nursing pre-armed with moral concepts and viewpoints. His view seems to be that these are sufficient to characterise the moral problems faced by nurses – such as those referred to so far in this book. Framing moral problems in terms of moral principles merely obscures these problems behind a mass of jargon.

An 'unjust' conception of justice (Okin, 1987; Tronto, 1987, p. 248).

This charge asserts that the principle-based approach is one which has the concept of justice at its heart, and that this is somehow an unreliable concept.

This assertion that the approach relies heavily on justice is a fair one, since, of course, the principle of justice figures as a level-three moral principle. Also, it may be said that a reliance on justice is implicit throughout the framework since, in its application, equals are to be treated equally in that the competent, autonomous decisions of any moral agent should be respected.

It should be said that the concept of justice is one which has long been at the centre of moral philosophy. Plato, Aristotle and (as seen earlier), more recently Rawls and Nozick have discussed the concept at length. Note that the philosophers just listed are all male and that, further, a more extensive list would include few female philosophers (see Baier, 1985). Suppose it is suggested that those philosophers who have influenced thought concerning justice develop their initial conception of what justice is on the basis of their experiences within the family. Such a suggestion is not implausible since Rawls, for example, sets out how the notion of justice derives from inter-actions within the family (Rawls, 1971, pp. 462–79; Kymlicka, 1990, p. 266). Suppose it is then argued, further, that the family itself is an unjust social institution. It may be said that the family is maintained by the subjugation of females and that this is manifested, typically, in an unfair division of domestic labour and maintained by economic disenfranchisement of fe-males (see Kymlicka, 1990, ch. 7).

Given acceptance of these two claims, it can seem plausible to query the legitimacy of the concept of justice which is con-sidered central to moral philosophy. This is so, it may be said, since that concept is based upon or derived from experiences of situations which are themselves unjust (namely, family experi-ences).

It should be added that in the care-based approach, a major and mutually exclusive division is asserted between so-called 'justice-based' or principle-based approaches to ethics, and care-based approaches (Alderson, 1990, p. 207). For our pur-poses, the principle-based view will be regarded as a version of a 'justice-based' approach, and only the familiar term 'principle-based' will be used henceforth.

A care-based approach

The care-based approach to ethics is very much associated with the work of Carol Gilligan (1982; also Noddings, 1984). Her views stemmed from a reaction to, and rejection of, a principle-based approach to ethics put forward in the work of the psychologist Laurence Kohlberg (1981, *The Philosophy of Moral Development*). Kohlberg proposed a theory of moral development upon the basis of inviting subjects to offer their views on various hypothetical moral problems. He claimed to identify six broad levels of moral thinking from his research data; further, he proposed that these form a hierarchy. At Kohlberg's lowest level of moral thinking, subjects reason entirely egocentrically; judgements concerning the rightness or wrongness of actions are based solely upon crude consideration of their perceived rewards or punishments. At Kohlberg's highest level of moral reasoning, subjects deliberate by recruiting 'universal ethical principles' (1981). Actions are morally right insofar as they accord with these principles and result from their employment in moral reasoning.

Gilligan voiced a serious, perhaps fatal, criticism of Kohlberg's claims. She drew attention to the fact that Kohlberg employed only male subjects when conducting the research upon which his conclusions were founded. Gilligan conducted research of her own, this time comparing the way female and male subjects reason about moral problems. Her conclusions include the claim that female subjects exhibit a 'care-focus' (The Caring Claim) in their moral reasoning, which is much less likely to be present in male subjects (see Gilligan, 1982, 1986; Kittay and Meyers, 1987).

In characterising the care-based view, Gilligan makes use of an example of a moral problem which Kohlberg set his subjects. In this example, the wife of a man, Heinz, is dying: a chemist has a drug which will save his wife, but Heinz cannot afford to buy it. Kohlberg poses the question, 'Should Heinz steal the drug?' (Gilligan, 1982, p. 26). An eleven-year-old male subject, Jake, apparently concludes that Heinz should steal the drug. According to Gilligan, Jake conceives of the dilemma as:

> [A] conflict between the values of property and life, [and] he uses that logic to justify his choice.

Gilligan goes on to say that Jake constructs the dilemma 'as an equation and proceeds to work out the solution'. The suggestion here is that Jake analyses the moral problem roughly in terms of competing principles, and attaches a weight to these. Since, in Jake's analysis, the life of Heinz's wife counts for more than the wrong done to the chemist, he reasons that it is right to steal the drug. For Gilligan's purposes, Jake can be seen as a representative of a principle-based view.

Jake's mode of moral reasoning is contrasted with that of another subject, Amy. Gilligan suggests that Amy's construal of the problem is entirely different; she conceives of the problem as a 'narrative of relationships that extends over time' (1982, p. 28) – The Caring Claim. She does not approach the problem by applying abstract moral principles to it. Amy, instead, considers the relationship of the people involved in the problem, and the effects on that relationship of Heinz stealing the drug (The Uniqueness Claim and The Emotions Claim). Also, Amy is reluctant to give a straight answer to Kohlberg's question (due to The Uniqueness Claim). Gilligan quotes Amy:

> If he [Heinz] stole the drug, he might save his wife then, but if he did he might have to go to jail, and then his wife might get sicker again, and he couldn't get more of the drug, and it might not be good. So, they should really just talk it out and find some other way to make the money.

Gilligan's proposal that there is a significant difference between the approaches to the problem by Jake and Amy seems a plausible one. Jake's analysis involves weighing general principles. Amy, in contrast, seems to focus much more on contextual factors (The Uniqueness Claim): both the problem and the 'solution' seem much less clear-cut for Amy than for Jake. Gilligan, of course, provides other examples in support of her claims to identify a 'different voice' in moral reasoning, but hopefully the example just offered gives sufficient indication of the nature of the 'difference' for our purposes.

As seen, Gilligan has suggested that Amy (and females generally) employs a 'care-focus' which is virtually absent in males. But what does this mean? What does The Caring Claim amount to? According to another care-based theorist, Noddings, caring for a person involves, crudely, empathic appreciation of the predicament of that person together with an appreciation of what is in the person's best interests (Noddings, 1984, p. 24).

We return to discuss Noddings' work later, but it should be said that nothing in her conception of care seems unique to females; surely males are capable of caring in the sense just outlined. But, more pertinent to our present purposes is the point that this conception of care is one which principle-based theorists themselves may claim to recruit. It might be suggested that the best way to determine how a person feels, or what is in their best interests, is simply to ask them. This seems a reasonable way to apply the principle of respect for autonomy or to consider how to implement obligations of beneficence. So, the mere presentation of a conception of what care amounts to does not yet help to articulate a care-based approach to ethics.

Indeed, as noted earlier, it can prove extremely difficult to characterise the care-based view, and often it is described, quite usefully, by contrasting it with a principle-based view (Brabeck, 1983, p. 37). For example, it can be pointed out that the principle-based view emphasises objectivity and detachment in moral decision-making. This is perhaps most apparent in the principle of justice itself which, as we saw earlier, is an entirely formal principle bereft of reference to any actual properties or characteristics of individuals. The other principles employed in the principle-based approach can also be said to be abstractions from particular situations or contexts. The principle of non-maleficence, for example, can be regarded as a general principle abstracted from judgements in particular situations that one ought not to inflict harm.

Further, an emphasis upon detachment can also be shown to be present in other views on moral matters. In the law courts, judges are employed to pass fair punishments upon offenders. The nature of such punishments is not left for those affected by the crime to determine. Also, it is often said that a person is too close to a situation to view it objectively. Perhaps situations where the parents of a child campaign for scarce resources to be allocated to their offspring count here. Even in so-called caring professions such as nursing a nurse may be criticised for being too involved with a client – for being insufficiently detached from the client (Brown, Kitson and McKnight, 1992, p. 39). So, on some views of morality – allegedly including the principle-based view – The Privileged View Claim is implausibly denied. In the care-based view, contextual factors and involvement in situations which are moral problems are each regarded positively.

With respect to notions of involvement in moral problems as opposed to detachment from them (The Privileged View Claim), again the care-based approach places heavy emphasis upon such involvement: the views of the participants in a moral problem have greater, not less, weight than those viewing the problem from a less-involved perspective. And, one's moral obligations, it seems, extend to those one is engaged with in a caring relationship, and for whom one has moral responsibility (see, for example, Gilligan, 1982, p. 19; Tronto, 1987, p. 249) (The Caring Claim).

In continuing to attempt to set out the care-based view, use will now be made of certain recurring dichotomies which proponents of the view make use of and find especially significant. (The author is indebted to Kymlicka [1990, ch. 7] for much of what follows.) The dichotomies are: public–domestic, objective–subjective, and hierarchy–web. In the discussion, the occurrence of the four claims ascribed to care-based theorists will be signalled as they arise.

Public–domestic

Friedman writes:

> [Morality] is fragmented into a 'division of moral labor' along the lines of gender ... The tasks of governing, regulating social order and managing other 'public' institutions have been monopolised by men as their privileged domain, and the tasks of sustaining privatised personal relationships have been imposed on, or left to, women. The genders have thus been conceived in terms of special and distinctive moral projects. Justice and rights have structured male moral norms, values and virtues, while care and responsiveness have defined female moral norms, values and virtues. (1987, p. 261)

The suggestion here, then, is that a distinction can be made between public institutions and private relationships; the former are described as largely male monopolies, and the latter are left to females.

Further, when making moral decisions in public life, it is considered important that these are just, or fair. This, it may be said, is manifested in the (claimed, or aimed for) impartiality of such judgements. Decisions which display favouritism or bias towards a particular group of individuals may be considered unjust since they do not display impartiality. The requirement that politicians reveal their business interests is evidence of this view; as is the obligation on health care professionals not to endorse the products of a particular manufacturer for no reason other than that they are produced by that company.

In marked contrast to the public domain, the domestic domain is conceived to be inhabited mostly by females. Decision-making in this context, it is suggested, is heavily influenced by family relationships (The Caring Claim). The notions of 'care and responsiveness' (Friedman, 1987) are alleged to be the characterising features of such relationships (The Emotions Claim). The detachment which is an apparent requisite of decision-making in the public domain is supplanted by a (literal) involvement with those affected by the relevant decision. The involvement referred to here is one which is bound up with the notion of caring: one is involved with family members since one cares for them (The Caring Claim and The Privileged View Claim).

While males in the public domain are concerned with individuals conceived of abstractly as citizens or consumers, females are concerned with individuals defined by their particular characteristics – the properties which are unique to individual persons.

Objective–subjective

We have noted that decision-making in the domestic domain involves phenomena such as feelings, emotions and intuitions (Nicholson, 1983, p. 93) and that these features of moral experience are viewed positively from the care-based perspective.

In the theory of knowledge (epistemology), objectivity is associated with truth and knowledge. Truth itself seems importantly bound up with objectivity: if a claim is true, it seems, it is true from all perspectives, so to speak. Further, its truth is open to be discovered. If a knowledge claim is true, it should be possible for another party to verify the truth of that claim. Think especially of knowledge claims made in the sciences here: such claims, it seems, must be open to be verified by scientists other than those who advance the claim. To give an example: imagine that a person claimed to have found a cure for cancer but that it could not be tested by anyone. Would that claim amount to knowledge that the person had a cure for cancer?

These points concerning the notion of objectivity can be taken to support the view that impartiality is a desirable feature of knowledge claims. An enquirer who simply seeks to discover the truth, it may be said, is more likely to succeed than an enquirer who has a vested interest in the success of a particular hypothesis.

The suggestion, here, is that objectivity and impartiality are associated with knowledge and truth. Subjectivity, on the other hand, is associated with lesser notions such as opinion and belief. These may be described as 'lesser' since there is a necessary connection between knowledge and truth – a person can only be said to know that a claim is true, if in fact the claim is true. However, no such necessary connection obtains between opinion and belief, and truth. It may be true that I believe that a claim is true, or that it is my opinion that a claim is true, without its being the case that the claim is in fact true.

Still further, phenomena such as emotions, feelings and intuitions are standardly regarded as subjective phenomena. If moral reasoning is supposed to aim at objectivity, then such data would not be considered relevant to the outcomes of moral decisions. Subjective data such as emotions and feelings are standardly thought to impede rational decision-making, and certainly not to enhance it. The distinction between 'objective' and 'subjective' phenomena is intended to distinguish data which are open to view, so to speak, from data which are not. To give an example of the contrast, it may be said that one's height is objective data since, in principle, it can be measured by anyone. By contrast, one's feelings or inner thoughts at a particular time can be described as subjective data since these seem accessible only to the thinking subject.

Proponents of the care-based approach typically claim that subjective data are essential components of experiences of moral problems, and hence that they should be taken into account in moral decision-making; such data should certainly not be omitted as irrelevant, or as an impediment to moral reasoning (cf. Gilligan, 1982, ch. 5). Alderson says 'Traditions in science and philosophy which mistrust emotion and intuition have to be overcome' (1990, p. 209). Her implication here is that moral problems have a subjective element which constitutes legitimate data in moral decision-making – namely, the phenomena of intuition and emotions. Positions in moral philosophy which regard such data as irrelevant are open to strong objection. That is to say, The Caring Claim, The Emotions Claim and The Privileged View Claim are highly plausible, and views which do not acknowledge the force of these claims are highly objectionable.

Hierarchy–web

Gilligan describes two ways of conceiving of moral problems, and employs the metaphor of a hierarchy to characterise one of the ways, and the metaphor of a web to characterise the other (1982, pp. 32–3, 48). The hierarchical view is one in which moral problems are surveyed from above, so to speak, looking down on them with 'detached objectivity' (Alderson, 1990, p. 210). Also, in this approach moral principles or rights take their place in a hierarchy of other principles or rights. Allegedly, a view of reasoning about moral problems from this perspective pays little or no attention to emotions experienced – rather like decision-making in the public domain as this was described earlier. Alderson suggests that Ethics Committees tend to adopt such an approach.

In the approach which is characterised by the employment of the web metaphor, subjects are conceived as being enmeshed in a web of relationships; subjects are alongside and involved with those experiencing the moral problem and this, in turn, generates a moral problem for the subject. Anyone towards whom one has responsibilities is, it is claimed, part of this web of relationships (Gilligan, 1982, p. 32); such individuals may include family members, clients and colleagues (The Caring Claim).

Before moving on to try to offer an assessment of the care-based view, it may be worth reiterating some of the main points that have been made. It was noted that Gilligan's work is generally acknowledged as the beginning of the articulation of the care-based view of ethics. She claimed to identify a 'care-focus' in the moral thinking of females. This is held to be distinct from, and superior to, an allegedly male mode of thinking which focuses much more on the weighing of abstract moral principles; the importance of cool, detached deliberation, and the exclusion of emotional responses to moral problems. The latter kind of position closely resembles the principle-based approach. So Gilligan's work aims to identify a 'different voice' (1982) in morality, one in which considerations of involvement in relationships, care and emotional responsiveness are accorded the highest degree of importance.

In an attempt to elaborate the care-based position, three distinctions which care-based theorists exploit have been discussed: public–domestic, objective–subjective, and hierarchy–web. These distinctions were exploited to articulate further the care-based view and to distinguish it from the principle-based view. With regard to the public–domestic distinction, this is supposed to indicate that the features of the domestic domain are highly important, and are unduly neglected in moral theorising. The objective–subjective distinction illustrates the neglect of subjective factors (for example, emotions) in ethics and indicates the great importance of these in the experience of moral problems. The hierarchy–web metaphor illustrates the differing approaches to ethics represented by principle-based and care-based theorists. Principle-based theorists, it is suggested, view moral problems from 'above' so to speak – from a position of detachment. Care-based theorists, by contrast, hold that the most important perspective on moral problems is that of those involved in the problem, in particular, due to the fact that moral problems arise out of involvement in relations with others.

Hopefully, then, the reader is clear that the care-based approach involves commitments to the view that moral problems are unique (The Uniqueness Claim); that involvement in certain relations is characterised by care (The Caring Claim); that moral problems are accompanied by the experience of emotions (The Emotions Claim); and that those involved in the particular problem have a privileged view of it (The Privileged View Claim).

Criticism of the care-based view

Recall that one of the primary aims of Gilligan's *In a Different Voice* (1982) is to identify a way of understanding and conceiving of moral problems which is importantly different from that arising from the principle-based approach. It has been seen in the last section that it is not implausible to suppose that in this particular respect Gilligan can claim to have been successful. But it needs to be emphasised that the mere identification of a 'different voice' in moral thinking is not by itself sufficient to motivate the wholesale adoption of that voice by nurses. Further argument is needed to show that the care-based position is preferable to the principle-based position.

It may be claimed against proponents of the care-based view that Gilligan's work makes, at most, a descriptive point: namely, that there is this particular 'care-focused' way of viewing moral problems. But, ethics is a normative enterprise. Its concerns are with how people ought to act or reason in relation to moral matters, not how they, in fact, do act or reason about such matters.

What is required, then, is a further argument to show that the care-based view is preferable to the principle-based view. This author is not sure whether an argument of such a nature can be provided, but in order to arrive at an informed judgement concerning the debate between the two positions, it will prove necessary to set out certain criticisms of the care-based view. This task will be undertaken in the present section.

Of course, it may simply be *asserted* that the care-based is the one which ought to be adopted. But a supporter of the principle-based view might simply make the assertion that, on the contrary, it is the principle-based approach which ought to be adopted. In such a situation it is important that arguments are brought to bear upon the rival views. We have heard some of the worries which opponents (and supporters) of the principle-based view have about that position, and now it is time to consider certain worries which one may entertain in relation to adoption of the care-based view.

It should be said here that caring for clients is indeed a desirable trait in nursing staff and in health care workers generally. As will be shown later, however, saying that need not commit oneself to the adoption of the care-based view.

Criticism of the care-based view can usefully focus on the features identified in the introduction to this chapter and which were deployed in its characterisation; namely, the claims of Uniqueness, Caring, Emotions and Privileged View. Five objections are made here:

1. The first feature identified was the claim that moral problems are unique, and an objection to this runs as follows. There is a serious problem in emphasising the uniqueness of moral problems. Surely, as Seedhouse points out (1988, p. 94), when one is engaged in moral reasoning – especially as a health care professional – one would like to have some general rules to apply. (Recall the criticisms of 'act' theories in Chapter 2 above.) Otherwise, it seems, one could simply be reinventing the wheel on every occasion that one encounters a particular type of moral problem. If one regarded all moral problems as unique, unrepeatable and not, therefore, categorisable into types, then one would not be able to carry over anything learned as a consequence of facing one moral problem, to any other possible moral problem. In short, it seems that generalisations are things we cannot avoid doing if we want to learn from or benefit from our experiences. And further, it seems actually useful – perhaps necessary – to have a set of general moral rules or principles which form the starting point of one's deliberations about moral matters. Hence, The Uniqueness Claim seems objectionable.

2. Second, an objection to The Uniqueness Claim related to that just given can be derived from the work of Hare (1981, p. 21; 1952). He draws attention to a logical feature of moral judgements, which is their universalisability. To see how this feature of moral judgements is to be understood, suppose that when faced with a particular moral problem on a particular occasion, one judges that a certain type of action is the morally correct course of action to take – say, truth-telling. Hare points out that this commits one to acting in the same way in relevantly similar situations (hence, moral judgements are 'universalisable' to relevantly similar

situations). Otherwise, one's moral decision-making is simply arbitrary.

To give an example here. Consider that one provides a client with information concerning the whereabouts of a shop where he or she may purchase cigarettes, even though one would prefer the client not to smoke – it is to be assumed that one makes this decision on the basis of relevant considerations. Moments later, a client with the same type of medical condition and generally similar characteristics makes the same request. Given that one judged it right to give the first client the information she requested, it seems that one ought to give the second client the same information – for the same reasons. In fact, Hare's suggestion is that if one judges that in circumstances of a given type (call it type A) that a given course of action is morally correct (call the type of action type T), then one is committed to performing acts of type T in all situations of type A. Insofar as the care-based approach prohibits generalisations from situation to situation or context to context, it seems vulnerable to this objection from Hare – an objection stemming from consideration of the logic of moral judgements.

3. A third criticism focuses on The Caring Claim and The Privileged View Claim. According to The Caring Claim, caring for others generates moral problems. This, however, can easily be accepted by the principle-based theorist. What is more important in the care-based view is that The Caring Claim is supplemented with The Privileged View Claim: that those involved in moral problems have a more favourable view of them.

It may be said against this position that the care-based view thus encourages what might be termed 'moral bias'. By this it is meant the following. As we have seen, the care-based position places heavy emphasis on the connections between relationships and concern (The Caring Claim). It seems that the domain or extent of one's moral responsibility extends only to those with whom one has a relationship. The term 'relationship' here is of course intended to cover more than simply family relations; let us suppose that it stretches at least to clients, close friends, and perhaps further to casual acquaintances. On the face of it, at the very least, from the care-based perspective it would seem that one has stronger moral responsibilities towards those with whom one has relationships than to those individuals who lie outside of these. Consider now two examples of moral problems faced by individuals.

In the first example, a single parent has a limited budget to use for buying Xmas presents for his or her 10-year-old son. The son badly wants a pair of expensive, designer-label trainers costs which around £100. The parent is aware that this sum of money could go towards a disaster fund to prevent further deaths from a natural disaster which, let us suppose, has recently occurred (say, a flood in Bangladesh). What should the parent do? It is surely tempting to conclude that from the care-based perspective the parent should give the money to his son.

In the second example, suppose that a wife becomes aware that her husband, whom she loves, has committed a terrible crime – say, he has murdered a stranger. Suppose, further, that she is aware that her husband may kill again. Should she alert the police and turn her husband in? Again, it seems that from the care-based perspective she should not. She should seek to preserve her relationship with her husband. She has no moral relationship with his potential or actual victims since she does not know them.

Clearly, these are very crude examples of moral problems and they are open to the charge of underdescription. But, it would seem that, in principle, such details could be provided and so objections from the charge of underdescription could be avoided.

The objection being raised, then, is that moral judgements which issue from care-based reasoning exhibit a moral bias in favour of preserving existing relationships; and this may even include situations in which the lives of others are at stake – hence, the charge is that The Privileged View Claim is open to serious objection (see, for example, Tronto, 1987, p. 250).

An obvious way to defend the care-based view from the charge of moral bias is to say that, strictly speaking, subjects are supposed to have a relationship with all humans – that the web of relationships includes all humans. In fact, Blum asserts 'Gilligan means this web [of relationships] to encompass all human beings and not only one's circle of acquaintances. But how this extension is . . . to be accomplished is not made clear in her writings . . .' (Blum, 1988, p. 50; for textual support, see Gilligan, 1982, p. 57). The question of whether all sentient individuals are included in 'the web' also seems pertinent here.

It is not clear that this extension of the 'web' is at all a plausible move to make. It seems to be a straightforward misuse of the term 'care'. It may be said of me that I care for persons whom I am acquainted with and related to. It may be said of a nurse that he cares for those to whom he has a professional responsibility. But to say that a person cares for, say, a stranger in another part of the world – a part perhaps that the person has never heard of and has no conception of – seems such a strained use of the term 'care' as to constitute a misuse. To say that a person Smith cares for x (where 'x' stands for some person), seems to involve the claim that this is the result of some actual thought about x by Smith; this is implausibly denied in the response under discussion.

Also, recall that part of the appeal of the care-based approach stemmed from considerations arising from involvement in a caring relationship with a person. Again, this militates against applying the concept of care to situations in which persons do not even know of each other's existence. Hence, this third criticism of the care-based view seems a powerful one.

4. A fourth objection again focuses on The Privileged View Claim, and draws upon that derived from Hare and discussed in the second criticism just offered. Apart from the apparent logical properties or features of moral judgements, it surely is incumbent upon nursing staff not to be morally arbitrary in their moral decision-making. This seems a distinct possibility if the sole constraints on moral decision-making are those which issue from the care-based perspective (specifically that one's moral judgements are informed solely by considerations of care). It is, of course, required of nursing staff that they be accountable. As we heard in our discussion of the principle-based view, this

amounts to offering explanations of one's decisions and actions. Within the parameters of health-care practice, professional considerations constrain moral theorising. However, it seems that the sole explanation one can offer in support of moral decisions from the care-based view is that one's motives were sound ones – they were motivated by care and concern. But this is not enough. Care is important, but these considerations do not exhaust those relevant to moral decision-making in nursing practice.

Further, it is evident that more justification is required for moral actions than the mere fact that they were undertaken out of considerations of care. To see this, consider that a parent, out of care for their children, insists that they have a cold shower at 5.00 a.m. each morning; or that they go without food one day a week. When pressed for reasons, the parent says that their actions are sincerely motivated by care for their offspring. In the health-care context, suppose that a client is allowed to die against the client's wishes. Suppose, further, that the client's death results from a nurse intentionally omitting to resuscitate the client. (For discussion of such a case, see Curtin and Flaherty, 1982, p. 294.) The actions of the nurse may well be motivated by considerations of care – perhaps he or she thought the degree of suffering being endured by the client too great – but the further question of whether their actions are morally justified seems pressing.

5. A final criticism to be offered here is that the care-based line has within it an importantly damaging logical inconsistency (Blum, 1988, p. 57, 62). The charge of logical inconsistency is quite a straightforward one. Recall that in the care-based approach it is regarded as essential to consider particular moral problems as unique, context-based, nonrepeatable situations. Approaches which seek to make generalisations, or to make judgements based upon principles supposedly applicable to types of situations, are deemed inappropriate – due to The Uniqueness Claim. Put another way, moral claims which are supposed to carry universal applicability are ruled out on the care-based line. But, it is apparently claimed at the same time that the care-based approach itself is one which is applicable across a great many, perhaps all,

moral problems. The difficulty here is one common to theses which seek to exclude general claims. Evidently, in seeking to rule out general claims one makes a general claim – a claim applicable to a broad class of cases. It may be said that this logical difficulty can be accepted. But even if this is true, it seems to be being claimed that the care-based view is in fact a view which makes a general – dare one say universal – claim for its applicability. (The author is indebted to Blum, 1988, here.)

The above criticisms have mentioned three of the four main aspects of the care-based approach, but no mention has been made of The Emotions Claim. As will be seen later in this chapter, it is evident that this feature of moral experience ought not to be denied; however, it will be argued that principle-based theorists can allow this.

In summary, then, it can be pointed out that the care-based approach can be subjected to at least the above five criticisms and that most, perhaps all, of these seem to be powerful ones. Before we can begin to articulate a preferred position, two further tasks need to be accomplished. First, to set aside a claim that is both misleading and widely prevalent in the nursing literature; and, second, to try to address the criticisms of the principle-based line discussed earlier.

A common misconception: care is not the essence of nursing

One reason why nurse theorists may be highly sympathetic to recruitment of the care-based approach to nursing ethics, is due to wide acceptance of the claim that care is the essence of nursing (due, mainly, to Leininger, 1984, p. 5; but see also McKenna, 1993). Of course, it highly implausible to claim that caring is not justly considered an important aspect of nursing practice. It would seem that Benner and Wrubel (1989) are entirely correct to point to the primacy of caring in nursing. However, the claim that caring is of prime importance to nursing is distinct from the claim that care is the essence of nursing.

The present author has argued that care is not, in fact, the essence of nursing (Edwards, 1994c). The reason is quite straightforward. The term 'essence' has its origins in ancient Greek metaphysics – especially that of Aristotle (see, his *Metaphysics*, Bk.VII, in Ackrill, 1987, pp. 255–360). In brief, essences are characteristics which distinguish kinds of stuffs or things. Hence, the reason that, say, water, tigers and humans differ is that they are constituted by different essences: the essence of water is H_2O and that of humans and tigers would be given by their respective genetic make-ups. Hence, essences are characteristics which are unique to kinds of things or stuffs – for example, to biological kinds or groups such as those just mentioned.

To claim that care is the essence of nursing, is to claim that care is unique to nursing in the same way in which, say, H_2O is unique to water. Hence, it would be to claim that all and only nurses take part in the activity of caring. This is plainly not the case since many other types of people are engaged in activities which involve caring – examples include social workers, medical staff, vets and parents (cf. Cash, 1990). So, whilst it is correct to say that caring is of prime importance to nursing, or a central concern of nursing, to claim that caring is the essence of nursing is to misuse the term 'essence'.

For present purposes, then, any claim to the effect that since care is the essence of nursing, the care-based approach must necessarily be adopted, can easily be rejected. It is important to reiterate that to deny that care is the essence of nursing is not to deny that care is important to nursing. Hence, within the sphere of nursing ethics it could be proposed that approaches to this subject can allow a role for caring. Indeed, given the importance of caring to nursing, it seems plausible to hold that a general stance to nursing ethics should make room for care-based considerations. Of course, to say this is not to say that care-based considerations do not require supplementation. Before we can consider such a position, the criticisms raised against the principle-based approach now need to be addressed.

A defence of a principle-based approach

It was mentioned above that attempts in moral philosophy to defend one particular approach in preference to another raise considerable problems of philosophical method. For example, what kinds of considerations could be relevant? Apparently, in other disciplines if there is a dispute between two rival theories a test situation is devised and the theories evaluated in the light of the test situation. But how can approaches to ethics be subjected to tests? For example, suppose Smith claims that water freezes at zero degrees centigrade but Jones claims that water freezes at two degrees centigrade. Their respective claims can be put to the test. But it is not quite so easy to evaluate the merits of rival approaches to ethics. Certainly discussion of the application of the rival approaches to hypothetical or actual examples of moral problems can play an important role in such a process of evaluation.

Having drawn attention to this methodological worry, it should be said that, in this author's view, not inconsiderable progress can be made. We have seen that the care-based view suffers from a number of quite serious, if not fatal, problems. Further, we have seen certain criticisms made of the principle-based approach, and some responses to these criticisms will now be made.

Callous and uncaring?

The first charge voiced earlier was that the adoption of the principle-based approach by nursing staff renders their moral decisions callous and uncaring (see, for example, Alderson, 1992, p. 33). An example of the worry may help here. In discussion with some experienced, qualified nurses, the moral problems raised by caring for clients who are in need of pressure-area care were mentioned. Specifically, the nurses spoke of the difficult moral problem faced when a client who in the nurse's considered view is in urgent need of pressure-area care competently refuses such care. Two nurses – call them nurse A and nurse B – spoke of having recently experienced such a situation. The students had been introduced to the rudiments of the principle-based approach to nursing ethics and were familiar with difficulties concerning the relationship between respect for autonomy and paternalism.

Nurse A simply stated that as far as he was concerned, if a client refused pressure-area care, knowing the consequences of such a refusal, then the client's wish would be respected – as is required, perhaps, by the obligation to respect the autonomy of clients.

Nurse B's approach seemed to differ, in what seems to me to be an important way. This nurse said that he did not take the client's refusal at face value, so to speak. He (nurse B) tried to enter into a dialogue with the client, asking the client whether there was anything that he was concerned about. Having given the client the opportunity to mention anything that was of concern to him, the nurse then asked the client again if his pressure-area care could be carried out. Nurse B added that if the client still refused, then the obligation to respect the autonomy of the client should be respected.

At the time of the discussion, it occurred to me (and still, at the time of writing, it occurs to me) that I would prefer to be in the care of nurse B than nurse A. It did, indeed, sound as though A's implementation of the principle-based approach had '. . . a chilly, uncaring emphasis on respect as non-interference' (Alderson, 1992).

But, it seems wholly wrong to say of nurse B's approach to the situation that it was 'chilly' or 'uncaring'. In the approach, it seems plausible to claim that the obligations of beneficence and respect for autonomy are considered in a way *infused with care*. Even though, ultimately, nurse B may have decided to respect the competent, autonomous wish of the client to forgo his pressure-area care, this decision was made out of considerations informed by the principle-based approach and by adoption of a caring attitude towards the client. Ultimate weight is carried by principle-based considerations, though care-based considerations are not neglected as irrelevant (see also Blum, 1988, p. 55).

So, in response to the charge that the principle-based approach fosters a callous and uncaring attitude among nursing staff, it can be pointed out that the approach can be applied in a manner which is infused with a caring attitude towards clients (and, of course, colleagues).

Overly simplistic?

The second criticism described earlier, takes two basic forms. In the first it is claimed that implementation of the principle-based approach omits much of what is central to moral problems. This includes the emotional experiences, for example, frequently undergone by those engaged in moral problems (Gilligan, 1982, ch. 4 *passim*). The second 'overly simplistic' charge stems from Alderson's comment that in crude principle-based approaches 'morality' is '. . . reduced to two or three principles . . .' (1992, p. 33) one of which is given greater weight.

The first charge, here, can be answered by pointing out that adoption of the principle-based view need not entail disregard for phenomena such as the experiences of those undergoing moral problems. For example, in nursing ethics courses it can be extremely important to recognise such experiences as legitimate, and to allow room for the expression of them (cf. Edwards, 1994a). Also, it is extremely important to take into account that those undergoing a moral problem are likely to be experiencing psychological distress. As far as this author can determine, nothing in the principle-based approach is compromised by the adoption of such a strategy.

The second charge can be responded to as follows. It is not being claimed here that the principle-based approach provides an exhaustive account of morality. Rather, an apparently plausible and argued-for position in nursing ethics is being set out. If, ultimately, arguments can be shown to favour one view over another, then, yes the second view is taken to be better motivated. But, of course, this is what debate about moral matters involves – the provision of arguments and counter-arguments. Hence, this author sees no genuine charge to answer here.

Too complicated and jargon-laden?

The third objection arose from the charge that the principle-based approach is too complicated and jargon-laden, and was ascribed to Hunt (for example, 1994a, p. 4). In response to this objection, it can be pointed out that moral problems themselves are complex and hence that the level of difficulty lies in the subject matter itself and not the approach canvassed in the principle-based line.

Perhaps it may be countered that the real criticism is that the principle-based approach is *unnecessarily* complicated and jargon-laden. However, it should be evident that the theoretical terms which do the work in the approach can easily be translated into ordinary, non-technical language. Nurses (and clients) themselves appear to have little difficulty learning the rudiments of the principle-based view, so it is hard to see how the charge of being confusingly complex can be made to stick.

It may be recalled, also, that in Chapter 1 above it was claimed that the language of the principle-based approach provides nurses with a language within which to couch their explanations of their actions – as accountable professionals are required to do. It is a fact that all the academic disciplines which are relevant to nursing have their own technical vocabularies (think of sociology, psychology and human biology), and ethics is no different in this respect. Perhaps it is unfortunate that, often, such technical vocabularies are employed to baffle and intimidate those unfamiliar to a particular discipline. There is some truth in the adage that knowledge is power. But this is a much wider issue than can be covered in a nursing ethics textbook. And nurses, at this very moment, are being called upon to make moral decisions and to account for them. Hence, it seems entirely reasonable that nurses should make use of the vocabulary of the principle-based approach for the reasons set out earlier in Chapter 1.

An unjust conception of justice?

The fourth objection considered was that stemming from the charge that the principle-based approach is founded upon an unjust conception of justice (see, for example, Okin, 1987; Tronto, 1987). It can be agreed from the outset that most of the standard philosophical authorities on theories of justice are males. Further, it should be agreed that, presumably, most of these authorities lived in families, and perhaps it is the case that the domestic arrangements in these families reflected broader social prejudices which included sexism against females.

In some respects this is a peculiar criticism. Recall in our discussion of Gilligan's claims that it was pointed out that, at most, she provides descriptive points; and that further argument is required to compel us to adopt the way of thinking about ethics which is found in the 'different voice'. A directly parallel response can be made here. It can be accepted that those philosophers who have most influenced philosophical thought on justice were brought up in an unjust social institution – the family; and perhaps even in an unjust society. This seems especially true of Plato and Aristotle. In ancient Athens, females and 'slaves' were apparently denied any say in the affairs of the state.

However, this is again, at most, a descriptive point. It does not show the thinking of those philosophers about justice to be fatally flawed. It could even be suggested that the very injustice of the social arrangements which surrounded them prompted them to think carefully about what justice consists in.

Further, it should be said that the formal definition of justice offered by Aristotle which we considered above, in fact helps to show just why, say, sexism is unjust. In sexist societies or social institutions, individuals are discriminated against upon the basis of their possessing characteristics which are not relevant from the moral perspective – namely, their sex, the colour of their eyes, how tall they are, and so on. So again, the principle-based view can be defended against the present objection.

In the discussion of the care-based view earlier in this chapter, it was noted that the view can usefully be explicated by reference to at least three dichotomies, that between the public and the domestic domain, between objectivity and subjectivity, and between the metaphors of hierarchy and web. The last two dichotomies contain certain elements which are in tension with the principle-based approach and so this needs to be addressed.

The objective–subjective dichotomy raises differences in emphasis between the care-based and principle-based views. As noted earlier, a supposed merit of the care-based position is that so-called subjective phenomena are taken into account in moral decision-making. The implicit objection is that the principle-based approach devalues such phenomena or regards them as impairments to moral decision-making.

It should be pointed out that the principle-based line can be applied in such a way as to acknowledge the importance of subjective phenomena such as emotions. As was recognised above, very frequently moral problems are accompanied by experiences of psychological distress. It is important to discuss the way it feels to be engaged in a moral problem. This can be of great educational benefit in addition to helping nurses learn from their experiences of moral problems in practice. So, it cannot be said that a principle-based approach must necessarily exclude all reference to subjective phenomena.

It may be countered that the fundamental difference between the two approaches is the weight attached to subjective phenomena. It is accurate to state that in the principle-based line great emphasis is attached to the employment of reason and informed debate about moral problems. These are associated with what can be termed objective enquiry. Reasons for holding a position are requested, examined, defended and either retained or rejected. This kind of procedure for evaluating between incompatible claims is common (essential?) to all academic disciplines. Proponents of the principle-based view argue that these types of constraints on theorising are extremely valuable. Plausibly, one is in a better position to assess the force of a case when one has heard the arguments for and against it.

It seems that proponents of the care-based line wish to pit against this picture of rational debate, a position in which there are no constraints in disputes about moral matters. If reason is not a constraint in moral debate, then there can be no moral arguments and each position is as legitimate as any other. This is a view known as moral subjectivism. Some find this position attractive, but it is easily shown to be vulnerable to extremely serious objections (see, especially, Midgeley, 1991).

To give a brief indication of why moral subjectivism may be thought objectionable, recall that for such a theorist any moral view is as legitimate as any other. Suppose, now, one person claims it morally right to torture children for sexual gratification, and another person disagrees. For the moral subjectivist, there is no further discussion which can take place here: matters of right and wrong are simply matters of individual judgement. There are more technical and adequate objections to the position than that those just offered (Midgeley, 1991; Edwards, 1990). But, hopefully, the reader can see the danger in moral subjectivism and in positions which deny a role for reason in moral debate. The suggestion being that this is a danger into which the care-based position seems to fall.

It can be repeated again that a position which denies a role for reason in moral debate is not really one which accountable professionals can adopt and hope to meet their professional obligations. These require nurses to offer reasons in support of their decisions and not simply to base their decisions entirely on emotional grounds – though, it needs to be stressed, the importance of such elements of experience of moral problems is not being downplayed.

With respect to the hierarchy–web dichotomy, the claim here was that in the care-based approach moral problems arise among persons who are engaged in a 'web' of social relations. In contrast, the principle-based approach was said to be hierarchical in at least two ways: first, in that those making moral decisions were claimed to 'look down' upon those involved in the relevant moral problem; and, second, in that one or other moral principle is accorded a 'higher' position in the approach than other considerations.

Consider the first of these charges. In response to the first it should be pointed out that persons employing the principle-based approach in moral decision-making need not be conceived of as looking down upon the persons involved in the moral problem. For example, I may be a nurse sympathetic to the principle-based line and I may be involved in a moral problem – either during the course of my professional duty or in some other part of my life. Evidently, individuals who have moral decisions to make are also engaged in social relationships (of course, these include professional relationships too). So, a person who 'looks down' upon individuals involved in a moral problem is perhaps forgetting that they too are involved in the problem and so cannot consider themselves detached from it.

With regard to the second charge, it should be conceded that in the principle-based approach as it has been set out here, it has been claimed that the principle of respect for autonomy should be considered as the most weighty principle. But, it should be said that this position is not one randomly plucked out of the air, but rather one which has been motivated by argument. Hence, it would seem to this author that the second charge does not need further response.

In summary of what has been done so far in this chapter: the chapter began by identifying certain concerns which may be entertained about the principle-based view. A rival position was then considered – the care-based view – which was then subjected to criticism. This was followed by a brief argument against the claim that care is the essence of nursing, and a defence of the principle-based line from the criticisms voiced earlier.

Before moving on, it may be wise to reiterate certain of the factors which are being taken here to motivate acceptance of a principle-based view (though one in which certain subjective phenomena are recognised as legitimate) and rejection of a purely care-based view.

It was pointed out above that the attempt to show one approach to ethics to be preferable to another raises quite serious methodological difficulties. But it was suggested that these may not prove insuperable (see also Benjamin and Curtis, 1986, pp. 39–44). One way to assess rival approaches is to test them for internal consistency. Consistency, it can be said, is a constraint on any approach put forward in any subject matter. That is to say, it should be expected of any view that it does not contradict itself, and this can be described as a condition of adequacy on any approach. However, as we saw earlier, the care-based approach seems not to meet this condition of adequacy. It should be added that the principle-based line seems not to contain any internal contradiction.

A second constraint, or condition of adequacy, to which any approach in subject is that deriving from considerations of meaning: does the approach make sense? It can reasonably be proposed that both the approaches under consideration here satisfy this second condition of adequacy.

These last two conditions are uncontroversially applicable to all moral theories and approaches to health-care ethics. However, it seems plausible that the two constraints just described do not go far enough in terms of their applicability to nursing ethics. The reason is that any approach to nursing ethics must be compatible with the conditions which constrain professional practice. Hence, it seems that it would count against a proposed approach if it was not compatible with the professional obligations of nursing staff. It seems to me that the care-based view suffers from such an inadequacy. The reasons are those already mentioned. As seen above, the care-based view appears to lead to moral subjectivism, and this seems to be incompatible with the professional obligations which bind nursing staff. The clauses of the UKCC Code oblige nurses to act in certain types of ways – ways which seem easily characterised by the use of moral principles. Also, the care-based approach seems to encourage a case-by-case approach to nursing ethics. Again, as seen earlier, it is not clear that this is either possible or helpful. And, finally, for by now familiar reasons, the care-based approach appears not to require further justification for moral decisions other than that they were motivated by care. It was argued above that this is not sufficient justification for actions undertaken by accountable professionals.

A final position

In the light of the apparent flaws present in the care-based view, and the apparent strength of the principle-based line, we are now in a position to put forward in slightly more detail an approach to nursing ethics. This will still merit the title of being principle-based, but will acknowledge an important role for the kinds of considerations which are of concern to care-based theorists.

In discussion of the defence of the principle-based view, a position was referred to in which care-based considerations are regarded as legitimate. But, in a conflict between a decision motivated by such considerations and one motivated by principle-based considerations, it is the latter which win out (cf. Blum, 1988). Hence, the approach being canvassed here is one which is a combination of principle-based and care-based views, but in which principle-based considerations carry the greatest weight.

It was claimed earlier that although care is not the essence of nursing, it is still highly important to nursing. And, having rejected a care-based view, it is necessary to say a little more about the sense of the term 'care' that is being appealed to. Before doing this, it is useful to comment upon a definition put forward by Benner and Wrubel.

In their *The Primacy of Caring* Benner and Wrubel (1989, p. 1) write: 'Caring as it is used in this book means that persons, events and things matter to people.' By this definition, any event which can be said to matter to a person is thereby an event which the person cares about.

A serious problem with a definition such as this, is that it is far too general, and probably all cognitively competent humans can be said to care in this sense. For example, a person alone on a desert island might be said to care about events such as a high tide, and about things such as fruits or pretty pebbles. A person may be said to care about a soap on TV, or a traffic light changing to green. Certainly, nothing in the definition offered by Benner and Wrubel seems to render caring a phenomenon which should be of special interest to nurses. On their definition it is probable that dogs, cats and perhaps even goldfish can be said to care since, presumably, certain types of events matter to members of these species (say, feeding times).

Perhaps worse, on Benner and Wrubel's analysis anyone can be said to participate in a 'caring practice' (1989, p. 5). Clearly, 'persons, events and things' (1989, p. 1) matter to professional footballers, academics, schoolchildren and to any cognitively competent individual.

So, it does not seem to be plausible to appeal to a sense of the term 'care' which is close to that defined by Benner and Wrubel. Perhaps a more workable understanding of what is meant by care can be derived from Noddings' work (1984). Noddings raises the point (1984, p. 12) that caring can be considered from two, perhaps three, perspectives: the perspective of the carer (the nurse); the perspective of the 'cared-for' (the client); and a neutral, third-person perspective (one taken by a bystander).

Also, she draws a distinction between 'natural' caring and 'ethical' caring:

● *Natural caring* arises 'In situations where we act on behalf of the other because we want to do so'. The example she offers is that of a mother caring for her child. This falls short of being ethical caring, she claims, since this maternal behaviour is 'natural'. In support of this, she points out that 'maternal animals take care of their offspring, and we do not credit them with ethical behaviour' (1984, p. 79). So, it seems that natural caring is more closely associated with a set of behaviours which are not undertaken as a consequence of conscious choice, but rather result from some innate disposition (perhaps one genetically grounded?).

● *Ethical caring*, Noddings suggests, 'occurs in response to a remembrance of the first'. The view seems to be that one becomes aware of what it is like to care and be cared for by virtue of being the recipient of natural caring, and by being moved to act in accordance with it. She speaks of a 'transfer of feeling' (1984, p. 80); that is to say, one acts in a caring manner to certain others due to the fact that one has experience of being cared for.

In summary of ethical caring, she writes:

> The source of ethical behaviour is, then, in twin sentiments – one that feels directly for the other and one that feels for and with that best self, who may accept and sustain the initial feeling rather than reject it.

The suggestion is that one experiences the initial urge, so to speak, to care, and one's 'best self' inclines one to act upon those urges rather than simply to ignore them.

If we apply this notion of ethical caring to the nursing context, in general, it may be said that persons enter the nursing profession out of acknowledgement of a desire to care for those in need of such care. Persons who do not enter a caring profession may recognise that others are in need of care but ignore their 'best voice', so to speak, and leave that task for others.

In addition to her points concerning the three perspectives on care, and the claimed distinction between ethical and natural caring, Noddings seems to commit herself to the view that the 'cared-for' person recognises that they are being cared for. For example, Noddings writes:

> [For] (A, B) to be a caring relation, both A (the one-caring) and B (the cared-for) must contribute appropriately. Something from A must be received, completed in B. (1984, p. 19)

Hence, it can be seen here that Noddings is claiming that the caring relation must be 'completed' in some way. Presumably, something must happen in B, and we may take it that this

means that B must apprehend that they are being cared for –
that they are involved in a caring relationship.

With specific reference to the question of how the term 'care'
is to be understood, Noddings proposes that caring involves a
'displacement of interest from my own reality to the reality of
the other' (1984, p. 14). Further, she asserts:

> Apprehending the other's reality, feeling what he feels as nearly as
> possible, is the essential part of caring from the view of the one-
> caring. (1984, p. 16)

And:

> Caring involves stepping out of one's own personal frame of refer-
> ence into the other's. When we care, we consider the other's point
> of view, [and] . . . his objective needs. (1984, p. 24)

On this view, from the perspective of the carer, caring necessarily involves appreciating the position of the cared-for 'as
nearly as possible', and considering and respecting the 'objective needs' of the cared-for.

Consider the four elements of Noddings' position which have
just been mentioned: the three perspectives on care; the natu-
ral/ethical caring distinction; the claim that caring relationships
are two-place relationships; and the tentative outline of just
what it is that caring amounts to.

First, it seems that Noddings is correct to point out that caring
can indeed be considered from the three perspectives she notes.
Evidently, a carer might think that their actions are caring, but
this might not be perceived to be so by the one cared for; nor
by witnesses from the third-person perspective. The example
given earlier of a mother who insists that her children rise at
5.00 a.m. and have a cold shower may constitute such a case.
From the nursing perspective, a situation in which a nurse
pressurises a client into undertaking painful exercise – say,
poorly practised physiotherapy – 'for the client's own good',
might also be relevant here: the nurse's actions are undertaken
out of care, but are perceived as uncaring, perhaps even cruel
by the client.

The distinction between natural caring and ethical caring
seems less plausible. It is not clear that caring is a universal

phenomenon. Many children are brought up in the context of a caring relationship with significant others, but many are not. It seems to follow from what Noddings says that those brought up in an uncaring home environment would not experience natural caring, and that this would thereby hinder – perhaps even prevent – their capacity to engage in ethical caring (see Hanford, 1994, p. 188, on this issue). It is not clear that this is a claim one could make solely on the basis of *a priori* reflection – independently of empirical evidence. Further, it may be pointed out that even if one has experienced natural caring by being on the receiving end of it, again it seems not to follow that one will thereby also engage in natural caring. Cases of child abuse are widely reported, and it is plausible to suppose that on at least some occasions such acts are carried out by persons who were themselves cared for.

The claim that satisfaction of the caring relationship necessarily requires a contribution from the cared-for, also seems far too strong. Evidently, it is possible to care for individuals who are unconscious in deep comas and also for individuals who are in persistent vegetative states. Also, as Noddings apparently acknowledges (1984, p. 14), it seems possible that one may be said to care for certain artefacts – a favourite vase and so on. Clearly, items such as these cannot contribute to the caring relationship. So, again, it seems Noddings' claims are far too strong here.

Although the elements of Noddings' views discussed so far have been subjected to criticism, it should not be concluded that her points are not valuable ones. In the present author's view, Noddings draws attention to important features of the phenomenon of caring, but, as just seen, it seems that her conclusions are too strong. In weaker form they may have much greater plausibility.

With respect to Noddings' claims concerning the characterisation of caring, we may recall that she mentions 'interests' and the necessity to consider matters from the perspective of the cared-for – 'as nearly as possible'. This seems highly plausible. The suggestion is that in caring for another, one places oneself as closely as possible in the position of the person cared for, and tries to assess the situation from their point of view. As Noddings hints, metaphysically it is not possible to do this since one cannot literally step inside another person's head and see the world exactly as another person sees it. But, when one is engaged in caring for another it seems something like a necessary condition that one at least consider what the best interests of the person cared for may be. Further, the carer is obliged to act upon such an assessment.

On such a view, caring for unconscious clients amounts to considering the person's plight as much as possible from the perspective of the unconscious person, and acting upon what are judged to be the best interests of the person. One obvious and sensible way to try to determine just what the interests of a client are, is to ask the client. One might do this simply by spelling out the options available to the client in terms which the client can make sense of. This is simply a caring application of the principle of respect for autonomy. Of course, if the client is unconscious, one needs to consider the client's perspective on the client's behalf without the benefit of the client's own views.

Given this modest, fairly crude but hopefully plausible proposal on just what caring might be thought to include, let us return to the saga of nurse A and nurse B.

It was suggested above that nurse B's implementation of the principle-based approach appeared to be tempered, or infused with care: relevant moral principles are applied but in a caring manner. By contrast, nurse A's application of the principles did appear to display the chilly, uncaring aspect which Alderson (1992, p. 33) detects in principle-based approaches.

It should now be possible to try to fill out just what is meant by the claim that the principle-based approach can be implemented in a way which is infused with considerations of care. In the nurse A/nurse B example, nurse A simply informs the client that they are in need of pressure-area treatment at that time, and asks if this is acceptable to the client. This, it may be said, amounts to respecting the autonomy of the client. Since the client refused the treatment, nurse A leaves the client alone – again, a response ostensibly grounded in respect for autonomy.

Nurse B handles the situation differently. Although he recognises and is ultimately prepared to respond to obligations to respect autonomy, he considers the interests of the client.

Recalling Noddings's expression 'as nearly as possible', it is evident that if the client's pressure areas are neglected, then tissue damage will inevitably occur. So, the client's response at least jars with what would appear to be their best interests; that is, even when an attempt is made to consider what these may be from the perspective of the client. This mismatch between the nurse's judgement of what is in the client's best interests, having considered the situation from the perspective of the client, and what the client says (their refusal of treatment), prompts nurse B to take the interaction into another phase. He invites the client to discuss the fears, emotions and reasons behind their refusal of treatment. Having been given the opportunity to discuss these, and having been given a sympathetic explanation of the point of pressure-area care, the client agrees to have the treatment. This is a much more desirable way to implement a principle-based approach to nursing ethics. And the expression chosen here to characterise the approach is that the principles are implemented in a manner which is infused with care.

Finally, could this position of a principle-based line infused with care help in relation to the difficulties raised by consideration of suicidal clients? Regrettably, it would seem that it cannot. This is due to the fact that, in the position, although the principle-based line is implemented in a way which is infused with care, it remains the case that principles bear ultimate moral weight. Hence, in interactions with suicidal clients, the principle-based approach infused with care would entail broaching the encounter in a way analogous to the approach of nurse B in the last example. That is, the nurse ought to consider the client's position and try to engage the client in discussion of the feelings and so on, which prompt the suicidal intentions. It should again be stressed that this is a somewhat uncomfortable conclusion to draw.

6 *The supererogatory nurse*

In this final chapter, the discussion is focused once more upon the moral principles discussed in this book. Although the discussion is somewhat abstract, it is an example of the way in which the principle-based approach can be utilised to structure issues within nursing ethics, and to aid clear thought about them. The chapter begins by employing the principles to help to distinguish ordinary from extraordinary moral standards. This will then help to identify a class of actions which can be described as supererogatory (roughly, as will be seen, these are actions which are for the benefit of others, but which expose the actor to significant risk of harm). The question of the extent to which nurses can be said to be called upon, or even obliged to undertake such actions, will then be considered.

What are supererogatory acts?

Beauchamp and Childress (1989, pp. 366–7) suggest that a distinction may be drawn between ordinary and extraordinary moral standards. They indicate that 'everyone' is bound by ordinary moral standards; but, they add, it is not the case that everyone is bound by extraordinary moral standards. But how could a distinction between ordinary and extraordinary moral standards be set out?

One way to do this is to recruit the four principles discussed earlier in the present volume. For example, it can be claimed that the principles of respect for autonomy, nonmaleficence and justice structure the obligations of ordinary moral standards, but that these are buttressed by additional obligations of beneficence in the case of extraordinary moral standards. It is worth stressing that these principles generate fairly minimal obligations. These are, of course, obligations to respect autonomy, not to harm others and to deal with others fairly.

156

The more demanding obligations generated by the principle of beneficence do not appear to feature among ordinary moral standards. It is considered morally acceptable to eat meat, to ignore homeless people, and to ignore the plight of persons in poor countries.

In ordinary standards, a distinction is made between harming someone by omitting to help them, and harming someone by actively hurting them. Hence, although by ordinary moral standards, it seems, it is acceptable to walk past a person in need of financial aid (a person who is homeless and hungry let us say), it is not considered acceptable to strike such a person.

It might, though, be suggested that *even in ordinary morality* there is, in fact, an obligation to help the person in dire financial need – say, a homeless and hungry person. This amounts to the claim that it is widely considered a moral wrong not to help such a person. On such a view, it is held that some obligations of beneficence do feature in ordinary moral standards. This proposal sounds much too strong to the present author, but suppose that it is accepted.

Even if it is conceded that the obligations generated by the principle of beneficence do feature among ordinary moral standards, it may be pointed out that the extent of its application is extremely limited. For example, whilst there is a strong obligation not to harm others (by ordinary moral standards), there do appear to be limits to the obligations generated by beneficence.

By ordinary moral standards, the principle of beneficence does not appear to generate an obligation to act in ways which will benefit others if acting in such a way results in harm (or deprivation) to the actor. Hence, although it may be argued that by ordinary moral standards one is under an obligation of beneficence to the person who is homeless and hungry, it is unlikely to be maintained that one is obliged to give to the person to the extent that this will result in some suffering to oneself or to one's dependents. So, even if in ordinary morality it is the case that obligations of beneficence are recognised, these appear to be extremely limited, or weak.

Actions which are done in accordance with extraordinary moral standards are termed 'supererogatory' by Beauchamp and Childress (1989, pp. 366–7); such acts ' . . . are undertaken for the welfare of others beyond what obligation requires'. That is to say, such acts go beyond what is required by ordinary moral standards. Hence, a person who did act in ways which are for the benefit of others but which expose the actor to harm, or significant risk of harm, would be said to undertake supererogatory acts.

A person who acted in a way which was for the good of another person but which resulted in harm to themselves or their dependents, could plausibly be described as acting in accordance with extraordinary moral standards. By ordinary moral standards, such sacrifices do not seem to be morally obligatory.

It should be added that a fairly rough distinction can be made between actions which exemplify what Beauchamp and Childress term 'low-level supererogation', and what they term 'high-level supererogation' (1994, p. 485). An action which exhibited low-level supererogation would, presumably, be for the benefit of others but would expose the actor to low risk of harm, or low levels of harm. An act of high-level supererogation, obviously, would also be for the benefit of others, but would run a high risk of harm to the actor.

So, it seems possible to make out the distinction between ordinary and extraordinary moral standards by invoking the four principles. Further, as we have seen, making the distinction in this way makes possible the characterisation of supererogatory acts.

To whom do nurses have obligations?

As noted previously in Chapter 2, a distinction can be made between professional obligations (and duties) and moral obligations (and duties). By entering into the nursing profession, nurses take on certain professional obligations. These are stated in the UKCC Code (UKCC, 1992): nurses have obligations to respect confidentiality, the religious beliefs of patients and so on.

In addition to these professional obligations, it is plausible to hold that nurses are under certain moral obligations. It can be suggested that nursing is not the kind of occupation which people enter into simply for the financial rewards; rather, nursing is entered into by persons who, by and large, want to help others – want to do good. In chapter 1, we considered Seedhouse's (1988, p. xvii) claim that work for health is a moral endeavour. This is because health work involves striving towards an end which is deemed to constitute a 'good'; namely, the aim is to improve the health and develop the autonomy of those who are patients and clients.

So, nurses are certainly under professional obligations (as set out in the UKCC Code) and, if work for health is a moral endeavour (as it can plausibly be regarded), then nurses would seem to be under certain moral obligations. But to whom do nurses have these obligations? At least seven groups and individuals may be identified.

1. *Other nurses.* Clauses 13 and 14 of the UKCC Code indicate that nurses have professional obligations to their fellow nurses. Clause 13 states that nurses are under an obligation to have regard to the 'health and safety' of their colleagues, and clause 14 states a professional obligation to help one's colleagues ' . . . to develop their professional competence' (UKCC, 1992).

   The professional obligation to have regard to the workload of one's colleagues has its moral foundation in the principle of nonmaleficence; and the obligation to help colleagues may plausibly be said to have its moral foundation in the principle of beneficence.

2. *Clients and their relatives.* Professional obligations to promote the well-being and autonomy of clients and their relatives are indicated in clauses 1 and 5 of the UKCC Code. The moral foundations of these professional obligations would seem to lie in the moral principles of beneficence and respect for autonomy.

3. *Other health care professionals.* Clause 14 of the UKCC Code indicates professional obligations to assist other members of the health care team. Again, it can be said that the moral foundation of this obligation lies in the principle of beneficence.

4. *The general public.* The UKCC Code states that nurses are bound by a professional obligation, '[To] serve the interests

of society [and to] act in such a manner as to justify public trust and confidence' (UKCC, 1992). Presumably, this professional obligation has its moral foundation in the principle of beneficence. It is necessary that patients trust nurses so that they will cooperate in treatment regimes and give relevant information to aid diagnosis and so on (family history of the relevant disorder, for example).

5. *Themselves?* A question mark is placed here due to unclarity surrounding what could be meant by such an obligation. Minimally, perhaps it denotes an obligation to be physically and mentally fit enough to perform one's professional duties. But construed in such a way it suggests that this obligation only holds because it is instrumental to the well-being of clients; that one is only obliged to stay fit and healthy so that others may benefit from one's state of health. Construed differently, it may be held that one owes it to oneself to have a minimally decent standard of living with sufficient material comforts.

6. *Their dependents.* It is a view widely held among nurses and other moral agents that they have moral obligations to their dependents; and, further, that these are weightier than obligations to strangers. Again, the moral foundations of such obligations appear to be the principles of beneficence and nonmaleficence. The relevance of beneficence here seems self-evident: one is under an obligation to act in ways which will benefit one's dependents.

   With respect to nonmaleficence, suppose one loses one's position as a consequence of drawing attention to poor standards of client care. This may result in being unable to provide basic necessities for one's dependents, and it may be concluded by some nurses that they should keep quiet about their concerns (see, for example, Tadd, 1991; Hunt, 1994b).

7. *Their employers.* Curtin and Flaherty (1982, p. 154) suggest that these are two-fold. First, to practise as a competent professional; that is, to practise in accordance with the standards set out by the nurse's professional body – the UKCC of course. Second, to be involved in the management of the institution to some degree. Curtin and Flaherty point out that some nurses explicitly have such a role – for

example, nurse managers. But other nurses have such a role only implicity, by their day-to-day decision-making; for example, concerning how best to use resources such as linen, sterile dressings and so forth. One might usefully add a third obligation which nurses may plausibly be said to be bound by; namely, an obligation not to use health care resources wastefully.

In the case of item 7 above, it seems reasonable to regard all three of these obligations as professional obligations; but what is their moral foundation?

Recall the claim referred to earlier that work for health is a moral endeavour – it involves working to promote a good; the good of restoring health or fostering the autonomy of clients. These considerations remind us that the moral foundation of health care work involves (at least) the principle of beneficence. It is the case that health care should result in good for clients (even if on occasion it does not). Also, the principle of nonmaleficence is of central importance. The very least one would expect of work for health is that it does not result in harm to clients. The benefits they obtain should outweigh any harms they may suffer (say, in undergoing surgery).

So, presumably, the point of health care institutions is to work for health, and to make possible the conditions under which nurses (and others) can work to benefit others – where they can carry out the obligations generated by the principle of beneficence. This suggests that nurses' obligations to their employers (and colleagues) and to the institutions in which they work, are only legitimate obligations in so far as they contribute to the general aim of making people well. So, although nurses are under an obligation not to squander health care resources, they are not under an obligation to be so frugal with health care resources that client care suffers. In other words, the obligations nurses have towards their employers should not be permitted to overshadow the more fundamental obligations of the nurse; these being directed towards the client. This point is worth labouring a little since the overall aim of the nurse's obligations to her employers can be lost sight of. It can seem that being frugal with resources – an obligation to the nurse's employers – can outweigh an obligation to benefit clients. But it should be clear that the obligations to clients are more fundamental since the obligations to employers and institutions only exist because of the obligations to clients. This ordering of the obligations of nurses is, in fact, required by the UKCC (1989 'Exercising Accountability').

Do nurses undertake supererogatory acts?

Having offered a (fairly rough) criterion of what constitutes a supererogatory act, and having identified the parties towards whom nurses can be said to have obligations, it can now be asked whether nurses do, in fact, undertake supererogatory acts.

Consider the following scenarios:

1. A ward manager, Jim Smith, in mental health nursing is coming towards the end of a difficult shift. The work has been particularly hard today, not least due to there being two new staff members who, through no fault of their own, have needed close supervision. Further, there have been two clients admitted to the ward during the shift, and these proved to be more complex than is usual. A third client is expected to be admitted at 3.30 p.m., and Jim is due to complete his shift at 3.00 p.m., having begun at 7.00 a.m.

   At 2.30 p.m., Jim is informed that his colleague, June Brown, who is due to take charge of the ward at 3.00 p.m. is too ill to come into work. Jim's manager asks him to work 'an extra hour' whilst he tries to arrange to cover Jim's ward. Jim has arranged to collect his children from school at 3.30 p.m. and it is too late to arrange for someone else to meet them. In any event, why should he even consider doing this?

   Jim refuses to stay beyond 3.00 p.m. – though he feels guilty about this. A few minutes later, Jim's senior manager rings again. He sounds desperate and informs Jim that there is absolutely no means of covering Jim's ward between 3.00 and 4.00 p.m. Could Jim please reconsider? Think of the overtime payment he would receive. Jim now capitulates: not due to financial considerations, one hour's overtime is very little anyway, but he feels that he cannot leave the ward without knowing that cover has been confirmed; this would leave the new staff members in a vulnerable position, and the clients on the ward may be affected also. Of course, the situation is made more complicated by the fact that a further client is expected at 3.30 p.m.

What Jim has to do now though – and quickly – is to try to arrange for someone to collect his children. Fortunately, his partner is able to go to collect the children, despite the short notice. She is not happy about this change of arrangements, however, and she makes this clear to Jim. They had agreed that she would have that afternoon completely free so that she could complete an assignment for a course which she is studying.

As promised by Jim's manager, a replacement is found by 4.00 p.m. In spite of this, Jim does not eventually leave the ward until almost 4.30. His replacement is not familiar with the clients on the ward, and the client due for admission at 3.30 arrived instead at 4.00 p.m. Jim felt obliged to stay at least until the initial disruption caused by a noisy new client had subsided a little, and until his replacement had been given a very basic guide to what had been happening on the ward that day, and what to look out for during the next eight hours.

2. The second scenario arises in a busy accident and emergency unit. A client with a superficial head wound and various other bumps, bruises and grazes enters the unit and asks to receive attention. He is asked to sit down and informed that he will be attended to as soon as possible. It is evident that the client has been drinking. He becomes tired of waiting and exhibits extremely aggressive behaviour. He threatens to attack another client sitting nearby. A nurse, Ann Baird, asks the violent client either to leave the unit or to be more patient. The client then physically assaults the nurse with a blow to the face. A struggle ensues. Whilst one nurse calls hospital security staff, others try to free Ann Baird from the grip of the client; they too receive some kicks and blows from the client. Eventually, he is overpowered and the police remove the client from the unit.

An alternative scenario involving a risk of violence to a nurse is the following. David Jones works in a community home, and six persons with quite serious learning difficulties live in the home. One of the residents, Jamie, has extremely poor standards of personal hygiene. Further, Jamie resolutely refuses to have a bath, or even a wash. If efforts are made to press Jamie into having a wash, he becomes extremely aggressive. Over the years, a number of behaviour programmes have been attempted to change Jamie's attitude to washing but none have succeeded. Jamie's personal hygiene has deteriorated to such an extent that he now looks dirty and smells of stale perspiration. David, other staff members and residents feel that efforts should be made to persuade Jamie to have a wash, but he simply refuses. Staff members and residents alike are not sure what to do about the situation. Some staff members argue that if it is Jamie's decision not to wash, then this should be respected. Other staff, and the other five residents, are less sure of this. They think Jamie should be coerced into having a wash. Eventually, it is decided that David should try to pressurise Jamie into having a wash – even though this is against Jamie's wishes. David is apprehensive about taking on this task as he knows that Jamie could become aggressive and he is a strong and powerful young man. In spite of this, David attempts to implement the course of action agreed upon by the staff group and the other five residents.

3. In their discussion of supererogation, Beauchamp and Childress refer to obligations to care for patients with dangerous, transmissable diseases – they refer to HIV (1994, p. 486). They query whether such obligations may legitimately be demanded of health care professionals, or whether undertaking such work should, more properly, be 'optional' (1994, p. 487; see also Johnstone, 1989, p. 337). Consider, then, the following case example.

    Sue Brown is employed in a special unit for the care of persons who are HIV-positive. As is well-documented (see last reference), there is only a very small risk of transmission of the virus to health care workers via, for example, needle stick injuries. In fact, the risk of acquiring HIV from a needle stick injury is believed to be around 0.3 per cent (see, for example, Schecter, 1992, p. 223).) Sue occasionally thinks about the risks of acquiring the virus during the course of her work, but she does not dwell on this for too long. Her partner, though, does harbour concerns about the risk of transmission and, from time to time, the fact that in the eyes of her partner Sue deliberately exposes herself to this risk, is a cause of tension between them.

4.   Simon Wilson is a Community Psychiatric Nurse and has an extremely heavy case load. At the last count, he found that he has responsibility for over 60 clients. Many of these need closer supervision than he can provide – there are only 24 hours in a day. Frequently, Simon finds that he works over 12 hours a day. For at least three of those hours he is generally not paid, since his managers refuse to pay overtime for them. He has since stopped even trying to claim payments for any extra hours he works. Simon has complained bitterly to his managers that he is overworked, and that his case-load is far too big. Recently, a client of Simon's physically assaulted a complete stranger; the assault, it seems, was attributable to a deterioration in the mental health of the client. The client had been diagnosed as suffering from schizophrenia and had not taken medication prescribed for him – he had not turned up for the last two appointments at which he would be given medication by injection. Simon felt responsible in some way for the assault on the stranger, and for the deterioration in the mental health of his client. With a smaller case-load, he felt sure he would have been better able to monitor his client's mental health and thus prevent the harms suffered both by his client and by the stranger.

Simon feels that his work dominates so much of his life that he has little time for interests outside of work. When he does return home from work he feels too exhausted to do anything other than watch TV and drink alcohol. He recognises that his lifestyle is stressful and extremely un-healthy, and feels exasperated that there seems to be no end in sight to his present situation.

Consider the predicament of the nurses in the above examples. Recall that loosely following Beauchamp and Childress we defined supererogatory acts as those which are for the benefit of others, but which expose the actor to significant risk of harm.

In case one, Jim Smith is in a situation which raises conflicts of obligations to colleagues, clients, his immediate managers at the hospital, his dependents and partner, and, perhaps also, to himself. In short, the obligations to clients, colleagues and hospital managers seem to conflict with his obligations to his family and to himself. Jim ultimately gives greater weight to the obligations to the first groups just mentioned than to the obligations to his family and himself. His actions, it seems, are for the benefit of others – specifically his clients and his colleagues, even though they have at least two undesirable consequences: they deprive him of the pleasure of collecting his children, and they cause strain in the relationship between Jim and his partner. Each of these consequences, especially the second perhaps, can be described as harms which Jim undergoes; harms which result from actions which are intended to benefit others.

In the second case examples, it seems that Ann Baird's actions do qualify as supererogatory if she recognises that it is likely that the client will become aggressive. Her action is for the benefit of others – not least the client himself – but is one which exposes her to risk of significant harm. The same can be said of the colleagues who go to Ann's aid: they are exposing themselves to risk of harm for the benefit of others – in this case, Ann and other clients. In this incident, the obligations to others are apparently given greater weight by the nurses involved than the obligations to themselves.

With regard to the scenario involving David Jones and Jamie, here again it seems that David's action can be classed as a supererogatory action. He is exposing himself to risk of physical harms for the benefit of others – for example, possibly Jamie, and certainly the other staff and residents. In this case example, David places obligations to others above those to himself.

In the third case example, it was suggested that Sue exposes herself to risk of infection during the course of her work. It should be said here that the actual probability of acquiring HIV during the course of her normal duties seems quite low (Schecter, 1992). But of course, although the probability of infection may in fact be extremely low, the level of potential harm is extremely high: Sue is exposed to a small risk of acquiring a life-threatening infection. If the risk of infection were low, and the potential hazard not especially harmful, then it seems unlikely that Sue's role could be described as one which involves the undertaking of supererogatory actions. But, as we have seen, the magnitude of harm to which Sue exposes herself, for the benefit of others, is very great indeed. Hence, it does not seem implausible to claim that her role involves the undertaking of supererogatory actions.

The fourth example offered involved Simon, the Community Psychiatric Nurse. Due to an unreasonably heavy workload, he, it appears, is unable to fulfil quite basic obligations to himself. Specifically, he finds it impossible to carve out any leisure time for himself. This means that he cannot meet the obligations to himself in either of the two senses identified earlier: his work commitments prevent him from engaging in a life beyond work; and the same commitments seem to be driving him to a state of psychological ill health. Hence, he cannot meet the obligations to himself even when these are construed instrumentally.

Since, as in the previous examples, Simon's actions are motivated by an intention to benefit his clients, it seems again that his actions qualify as supererogatory acts.

It may be argued that none of the nurses we have considered act in ways which are describable as supererogatory. The reason why, it may be said, is that it is simply part of the nurse's role – the nurse's station, so to speak – to undertake the kinds of actions described in the examples just offered (see, for example, Beauchamp and Childress, 1989, p. 369). Since nurses are paid for their work, it may be said, their actions cannot be described as supererogatory.

There are at least two ways of responding to such an argument. The first simply exploits the conclusion reached in Chapter 1 above, to the effect that there is an intimate, perhaps necessary, relationship between ethics and nursing practice. Since the actions of the nurses in our examples satisfy the criterion for classification as actions with a moral component, the fact that the nurses are paid for their actions does not affect the claim that they are actions with a moral aspect.

It might also be pointed out that in the cases we described, the intentions of the nurses are uniformly to act in ways which benefit their clients and which expose themselves to certain harms. These considerations themselves seem to suggest that their actions meet the criterion of supererogatory acts put forward by Beauchamp and Childress (1989, p. 367) and described above. This is the case, it appears, even if they receive payment for such actions.

In addition to these last two points, as indicated by Beauchamp and Childress a distinction may be proposed between 'ordinary role obligations and extraordinary self-imposed standards' (1989, p. 369). Thus, consider a nurse who is placed in a situation such as that faced by Jim, but who responds differently. Suppose this nurse simply refuses to stay on beyond her official span of duty (it can be imagined that she has stayed on previous occasions but has decided that enough is enough). It can reasonably be supposed that the most one's ordinary role obligations require one to do is to work the number of hours one is contracted to work – perhaps with a small degree of flexibility on the part of the nurse. The standards which Jim imposes upon himself would seem to amount to extra-ordinary standards since, as seen above, they place obligations to clients above those to himself.

A parallel claim can be made in relation to Simon: his actions seem to exceed ordinary role obligations. Perhaps the actions of David fall into this category also. The reason is that he is exposing himself to significant risk of significant physical harm, and is doing so for the benefit of other parties (supposedly, including Jamie). It would surely be extremely dubious to claim that exposing oneself to high risk of serious physical injury could be regarded as an ordinary role obligation. Hence, it seems plausible to uphold the claim that the nurses in the example given above do act in ways which qualify as supererogatory.

Now, it may be said of Simon, and perhaps also of Jim, that he should simply try harder to obtain more support; that is, it may be said that there are simply insufficient levels of staff to meet the demand placed upon the mental health services in his area. To that extent, it can be seen that Simon's predicament is significantly different from that of Sue. Although it has been claimed that both Simon and Sue engage in supererogatory actions, Sue is at least able to meet the needs of her clients without working longer hours than she is paid to do. She, at least, has opportunities to meet obligations to herself, to her dependents (if any) and to her partner. Simon, it seems, is deprived of such opportunities. Perhaps, also, the same may be said to a lesser extent of Jim.

Let us focus a little further on the case of Simon. The reason for this is that many nurses seem to complain that they are being pushed further and further to work harder and harder, but with lower staffing levels. This is a complaint familiar to most people who come into contact with health care professionals, but it is not a claim for which empirical evidence will be provided here. The only evidence this author has is anecdotal, and is drawn from over three years of teaching nursing ethics to groups of student nurses and groups of qualified nurses.

Cases such as Simon's raise quite general issues concerning the very nature of the nurse's role, and concerning the nursing profession. For example, it may be that our considerations concerning the notion of supererogation have quite dramatic implications for the nursing profession – as can now be seen.

Nurses frequently point to the adverse consequences of drawing attention to bad practice or to inadequate standards of client care (the plight of Graham Pink is often cited [Tadd, 1991]). They fear being labelled a trouble maker, that their career prospects will be harmed (Hunt, 1994b; Brindle, 1991), and, worse, that they may lose their position. Such nurses may point to a conflict of obligations: obligations to clients on the one hand; obligations to themselves and their dependents on the other; or some other combination of conflicts of obligation.

What ought nurses to do in such situations? It can be seen that those who claim that nurses are indeed under an obligation to draw attention to poor standards of care (namely, those who expect nurses to act in accord with clause 1 of the UKCC Code), expect nurses to undertake actions which qualify as supererogatory. As we have heard, clause 1 of the UKCC Code (UKCC, 1992) indicates that nurses are under a professional obligation to '. . . act always in such a way as to promote and safeguard the interests and well-being of patients and clients'.

However, the extent to which nurses are obliged to act in accordance with this professional obligation may be unclear. For example, suppose that a nurse believes levels of client care to be below an appropriate level. Suppose, further, that the nurse acts in accord with clause 11 of the UKCC Code and reports to 'an appropriate person . . . circumstances in the environment of care which could jeopardise standards of care' (1992). Suppose, yet further, that having done this, no improvement in standards of care ensues (think of the case of Simon here).

What should the nurse do? Clause 1 of the UKCC Code seems to oblige nurses to do anything possible to ensure that the well-being of clients is protected. Hence, it appears that if the nurse takes this clause seriously (as they must do), then that nurse should become a 'whistleblower', and draw the attention of the media to the inadequate standards of client care.

But, in undertaking such action, it is evident that nurses may suffer some harms – both to themselves and to their dependents. The Department of Health's Management Executive have stated that breaches of confidentiality '[Will] always warrant disciplinary action' (Dept. of Health, 1993, clause 8).

So, a nurse who breached confidentiality in order to draw attention to poor levels of patient care would inevitably face disciplinary action, even if the breach is justified on moral and professional grounds (by virtue of clauses 1 and 10). If nurses are to take clause 1 of the UKCC Code seriously, it would appear to be the case that they are under an obligation to undertake acts which are supererogatory.

Nurses may point to the adverse consequences of (say) speaking out about low standards of client care or malpractice. Such acts are acknowledged by nurses to be for the benefit of patients, but are feared to have adverse consequences for the nurse concerned. Such acts do not seem to be obligatory by ordinary moral standards (since, by these one is obliged to do good only if it does not result in harm to oneself or one's dependents).

So, acts such as whistleblowing would appear to meet the definition of supererogatory acts defined above – they are for the welfare of others but go beyond what is obligatory by ordinary moral standards. It should be inferred, then, that nurses are not under an obligation by ordinary moral standards to draw attention to low levels of patient care, if in so doing they run a high risk of harming themselves or their dependents.

Should nurses be expected to take on the standards of extra-ordinary morality, and so perform acts which are supererogatory? Clause 1 of the UKCC Code (UKCC, 1992) seems to suggest that they should.

I do not propose to pursue this question in any depth, but the following three considerations seem relevant. First, it might be suggested that what are being balanced against each other are (a) actual harms presently being undergone by patients, versus (b) possible harms to the nurse and her dependents. It is not necessarily the case that any nurse who is critical of standards of care will suffer harms (examples of nurses who have include Graham Pink [see Tadd, 1991], and Roisin Hart [see Snell, 1992]). Also, it is plausible to hold that actual harms undergone count for more than possible harms in the kind of calculation envisaged in (a) and (b).

In response to this last point, though, it should be pointed out that the statement from the Department of Health quoted ear-lier seems to say unequivocally that *any* nurse who discusses confidential information beyond the context of the relevant hospital can expect to suffer some kind of harm – specifically, some form of 'disciplinary action'.

Second, given what has been said in this chapter on the subject of supererogation, a serious question arises as to the tenability of the position of nurses when their predicament is considered from the moral and the professional perspectives. From the moral perspective, the nurse's predicament seems especially problematic. A nurse who appreciates the moral dimension involved in caring for others must, minimally, rec-ognise obligations of beneficence. The desire to help those in need or to do something which is of benefit to people are among the main reasons why many people enter into the caring professions. Yet, it appears, in many instances a nurse may have to consider acting in ways which do not benefit clients, and which, in fact, may actually be harmful to clients. The examples of Simon and Jim present such cases: they weigh their obligations to their clients against those to themselves and to others. In our examples, they gave greater weight to the

obligations to clients – even though this is at considerable cost
to themselves. It has to be asked whether these are reasonable
expectations of individuals. In effect, nurses are being expected
to act in ways which count as supererogatory.

Consider also the nurse's predicament in the light of the Department of Health's position concerning breaches of confidentiality.
Hence, even if a nurse's actions are motivated by obligations of
beneficence, and even if the nurse has exhausted all internal
channels to campaign for improved standards of client care, the
nurse can expect disciplinary action for endeavouring to act in
ways which benefit others – clients and colleagues.

Even if such expectations of nurses are legitimate – the expec-
tation that they will undertake supererogatory actions – it
surely should be the case that nurses are forewarned about this
before they enter into the profession.

Considered from the professional perspective, the nurse's
predicament looks bleak – perhaps even untenable. The reason
is that their professional obligations by clause 1 of the UKCC
Code stipulate that nurses must act 'always'(!) in ways which
promote the well-being of clients. But what happens in situations such as that in which the hypothetical Simon finds
himself? If he is concerned about standards of care, the code
obliges him to 'report to an appropriate person or authority . . .
any circumstances in the environment of care which could
jeopardise standards of practise' (UKCC, 1992, clause 11). By
'standards of practice' here, one hopes that the UKCC do not
mean dismal or poor standards, but, at least, good standards
(standards which enable nurses to meet the obligations set out
in clause 1). In our earlier example, having alerted those within
the hospital – perhaps even the Department of Health (as did
Graham Pink) – to his concerns, what could Simon do? Either,
it seems, he could work unpaid overtime at considerable cost to
his own well-being. Or, he could alert parties outside the hospital (or Department of Health) to his concerns. But, as we have
seen, if he takes the latter course of action, he can expect
sanctions. If he takes no action, he is open to the charge of not
practising in accordance with professional standards as set out
in the UKCC Code. It would seem that if this diagnosis of the
position of nurses such as Simon is accurate, then the position
of the nursing profession in untenable. Nurses cannot act in

accordance with the standards set out in their own code of conduct. (For policy changes which will ease this problem for the nursing profession, see Hunt, 1994a, pp. 144–5.)

The third, and final, comment to be made here in response to the points made above concerning supererogation is slightly less serious than the previous two comments, but still one worth making. Of course, one substantial difficulty with any proposed distinction between ordinary and extraordinary moral standards is that extraordinary moral standards will inevitably be defined only relative to ordinary moral standards. Obviously, if ordinary moral standards were more morally demanding, then what would be regarded as extraordinary would differ. For example, suppose it is obligatory by ordinary moral standards to give away all one's possessions (except those essential for survival) for the benefit of others – say, persons in extremely poor countries. In such a moral climate, supererogatory acts would be extremely morally demanding – perhaps they may involve actions such as giving up one's life for others. In any event, we have no choice at present other than to define extraordinary moral standards by reference to the standards of ordinary morality in contemporary Britain, and so need not pursue this last suggestion any further.

In conclusion, it may be said that nurses who refrain from drawing attention to low standards of client care due to fear of possible harms to themselves and their dependents, are acting in accord with ordinary moral standards; those who do not so refrain, perform acts which qualify as supererogatory. Clause 1 of the UKCC Code appears to require nurses to act in ways which qualify as supererogatory, as that term has been defined here.

It is regrettable to end a book such as this – as so often seems to be the case in nursing – on a negative issue such as that just discussed. However, if the analysis offered in this chapter of the nurse's moral and professional predicament is accepted, the negative conclusions seem to follow. One way in which a chapter such as this can contribute to a resolution of the difficulties for the nursing profession is, at least, to give a fairly clear articulation of just what the problem is. In my view, the principles outlined in this book help to do this, as they can help in other areas of nursing ethics.

Bibliography

Alderson, P. (1990), *Choosing for Children* (Oxford: Oxford University Press).

Alderson, P. (1992), 'Defining ethics in nursing practice', *Nursing Standard*, 6, pp. 33–5.

Aristotle, *Nichomachean Ethics* (trans.), Thompson, J. A. K. (1955), (Harmonsdworth: Penguin).

Aristotle, 'Metaphysics', in Ackrill, J. L. (ed.) (1987), *A New Aristotle Reader* (Oxford: Oxford University Press).

Baier, A. C. (1985), 'What women want in a moral theory', in Larrabee (ed.) 1993, pp. 19–32.

Bandman, E. L. and Bandman, B. (1990), *Nursing Ethics Through the Lifespan*, 2nd ed. (London: Prentice-Hall).

Barker, J. (1995), *Local NHS Healthcare Purshasing and Prioritising from the perspective of Bromley Residents* (Hayes: Bromley Health).

BBC (1994), *Hypotheticals* (London: BBC Publications).

Beauchamp, T. L. and Childress, J. F. (1989), *Principles of Biomedical Ethics*, 3rd ed. (Oxford: Oxford University Press).

Beauchamp, T. L. and Childress, J. F. (1994), *Principles of Biomedical Ethics*, 4th ed. (Oxford: Oxford University Press).

Benjamin, M. and Curtis, J. (1986), *Ethics in Nursing*, 2nd ed. (Oxford: Oxford University Press).

Benjamin, M. and Curtis, J. (1992), *Ethics in Nursing*, 3rd ed. (Oxford: Oxford University Press).

Bloch, S. and Chodoff, P. (eds) (1981), *Psychiatric Ethics* (Oxford: Oxford University Press).

Bloch, S. and Heyd, D. , 'The ethics of suicide', in Bloch and Chodoff (eds) (1981), pp. 185–202.

Bluglass, R. (1993), 'The case for supervision', *Nursing Times*, 89 (6), pp. 32–3.

Brabeck, M. (1983), 'Moral judgment: theory and research on differences between males and females', in Larrabee (ed.) (1993), pp. 33–48.

Brown, A. (1986), *Modern Political Philosophy* (Harmonsdworth: Penguin).

Brown, J. M. , Kitson, A. L. and McKnight, T. J. (1992), *Challenges in Caring* (London: Chapman & Hall).

Buchanan, A. E. and Brock, D. W. (1989), *Deciding For Others* (Cambridge: Cambridge University Press).

Burnard, P. and Chapman, C. M. (1988), *Professional and Ethical Issues in Nursing* (Chichester: John Wiley).

Camus, A. (1955), *The Myth of Sisyphus* (Harmondsworth: Penguin).

Capuzzi, C. and Garland, M. (1990), 'The Oregon plan: increasing access to health care', *Nursing Outlook*, Nov./Dec. , pp. 260–86.

Carr, B. (1987), *Metaphysics: an Introduction* (London: Macmillan).

Cash, K. (1990), 'Nursing models and the Idea of Nursing', *International Journal of Nursing Studies*, 27 (3), pp. 249–56.

Chadwick, R. and Tadd, W. (1992), *Ethics and Nursing Practice* (London: Macmillan).

Clark, M. (1977), *Practical Nursing* (London: Balliere-Tindall).

Clouser, K. D. and Gert, B. (1990), 'A critique of principlism', *The Journal of Medicine and Philosophy*, 15, pp. 219–36.

Culver, C. M. and Gert, B. (1982), *Philosophy in Medicine* (New York: Oxford University Press).

Curtin, L. and Flaherty, M. J. (1982), *Nursing Ethics: Theories and Pragmatics* (London: Prentice-Hall).

Dancy, J. and Sosa, E. (1992), *A Companion to Epistemology* (Oxford: Blackwell).

Daniels, N. (1985), *Just Health Care* (Cambridge: Cambridge University Press).

Department of Health (1991), *The Patient's Charter* (London: HMSO).

Department of Health (1993), 'Guidance for staff on relations with the public and the media' (Department of Health, London).

Dickenson, D., 'Nurse time as a scarce health care resource', in Hunt (ed.) (1994a), pp. 207–17.

Downie, R. S. and Calman, K. C. (1987), *Healthy Respect* (London: Faber & Faber).

Dworkin, G. (1971), 'Paternalism', in Wasserstrom, R. (ed.) (1971), *Morality and the Law* (Belmont: Wadsworth), pp. 107–26.

Dworkin, G. (1988), *The Theory and Practice of Autonomy* (Cambridge: Cambridge University Press).

Dworkin, R. (1977), *Taking Rights Seriously* (London: Duckworth).

Edwards, S. D. (1990), *Relativism, Conceptual Schemes and Categorial Frameworks* (Aldershot: Avebury).

Edwards, S. D. (1993), 'Formulating relativism', *Philosophia*, 22, pp. 63–74.

Edwards, S. D. (1994a), 'Nursing ethics', *Nurse Education Today*, 14, pp. 136–9.

Edwards, S. D. (1994b), *Externalism in the Philosophy of Mind* (Aldershot: Avebury).

Edwards, S. D. (1994c), 'Care is not the essence of nursing', *Edlines* (November), Royal College of Nursing, pp. 13–16.

Fairbairn, G. J. (1995), *Contemplating Suicide* (London: Routledge).

Faulder, C. (1985), *Whose Body is it?* (London: Virago).

Feyerabend, P. (1975), *Against Method* (London: Verso).

Frankena, W. J. (1973), *Ethics* (London: Prentice-Hall).

'Free to leave at any time', *Open Mind*, no. 52, pp. 7–10.

Frey, R. G. (1983), *Rights, Killing and Suffering* (Oxford: Blackwell).

Friedman, M. (1987), 'Beyond caring: the de-moralisation of gender', in Larrabee (ed.) (1993), pp. 258–73.

Fuller, S. (1988), *Social Epistemology* (Bloomington: Indiana University Press).

Gilligan, C. (1982), *In a Different Voice* (Cambridge, Mass.: Harvard University Press).

Gilligan, C. (1986), 'Reply to Critics', in Larrabee (ed.) (1993), pp. 207–14.

Gillon, R. (1985), *Philosophical Medical Ethics* (Chichester: John Wiley).

Gillon, R. (ed.) (1994), *Principles of Health Care Ethics* (Chichester: John Wiley).

Glover, J. (1977), *Causing Death and Saving Lives* (Harmondsworth: Penguin).

Green, R. (1976), 'Health care and justice in contract theory perspective', in R. Veatch and R. Branson (eds) (1976), *Ethics and Health Policy* (Cambridge, Mass.: Ballinger), pp. 111–26.

Hampshire, S. (ed.) (1978), *Public and Private Morality* (Cambridge: Cambridge University Press).

Hanfling, O. (1972), *Kant's Copernican Revolution* (Milton Keynes: Open University Press).

Hanford, L. (1994), 'Nursing and the concept of care', in Hunt (ed.) (1994), pp. 181–97.

Hare, R. M. (1981), *Moral Thinking* (Oxford: Oxford University Press).

Hare, R. M. (1952), *The Language of Morals* (Oxford: Oxford University Press).

Harris, J. (1985), *The Value of Life* (London: Routledge).

Honderich, T. and Burnyeat, M. (eds) (1979), *Philosophy as It Is* (Harmondsworth: Pelican).

Hunt, G. (ed.) (1994a), *Ethical Issues in Nursing* (London: Routledge).

Hunt, G. (ed.) (1994b), *Whistleblowing in the Health Service* (London: Edward Arnold).

Hussey, T. (1990), 'Nursing ethics and project 2000', *Journal of Advanced Nursing*, 15, pp. 1377–82.

Johnstone, M. J. (1989), *Bioethics: a Nursing Perspective* (London: Bailliere-Tindall).

Kant, I. [1785], *Groundwork of the Metaphysic of Morals*, in H. J. Paton (trans) (1948), *The Moral Law* (London: Hutchinson).

Kim, J. (1976), 'Events as property exemplifications', in M. Brand and D. Walton (eds), *Action Theory* (Dordrecht: Reidel), pp. 158–77.

Kittay, E. and Meyers, D. (eds) (1987), *Women and Moral Theory* (New Jersey: Rowman & Littlefield).

Kleinberg, S. S. (1991), *Politics and Philosophy* (Oxford: Blackwell).

Kohlberg, L. (1981), *The Philosophy of Moral Development* (San Francisco: Harper & Row).

Kuhn, T. S. (1962), *The Structure of Scientific Revolutions* (Chicago: Chicago University Press).

Kymlicka, W. (1990), *Contemporary Political Philosophy* (Oxford: Oxford University Press).

Kuhse, H. and Singer, P. (1985), *Should the Baby Live?* (Oxford: Oxford University Press).

Larrabee, M. J. (ed.) (1993), *An Ethic of Care* (London: Routledge).

Leininger, M. M. (ed.) (1984), *Care: The Essence of Nursing and Health* (New York: Slack).

Loehy, E. H. (1991), 'Involving patients in DNR decisions', *Journal of Medical Ethics*, 17, pp. 156–60.

Lyons, D. (1965), *Forms and Limits of Utilitarianism* (Oxford: Clarendon Press).

Macdonald, C. (1989), *Mind–Body Identity Theories* (London: Routledge).

Maclean, A. (1993), *The Elimination of Morality* (London: Routledge).

Mason, J. K. and McCall Smith, R. A. (1994) *Law and Medical Ethics*, 4th ed. (London: Butterworths).

McKenna, G. (1993), 'Caring is the essence of nursing practice', *British Journal of Nursing*, 2 (1), pp. 72–6.

Melia, K. (1989), *Everyday Nursing Ethics* (London: Macmillan).

Midgeley, M. (1991), *Can't We Make Moral Judgements?* (Bristol: Bristol Press).

Mill, J. S. [1863], 'Utilitarianism', in M. Warnock (ed.) (1962), *Utilitarianism* (London: Fontana).

Moskop, J. C. (1983), 'Rawlsian justice and a human right to health care', *The Journal of Medicine and Philosophy*, 8, pp. 329–38.

Nicholson, L. J. (1983), 'Women, morality and history', in Larrabee (ed.) (1993), pp. 87–101.

Noddings, N. (1984), *Caring: A Feminine Approach to Ethics and Moral Education* (Los Angeles: University of California Press).

Nozick, R. (1974), *Anarchy, State and Utopia* (Oxford: Blackwell).

Okin, S. (1987), 'Justice and gender', *Philosophy and Public Affairs*, 16, pp. 42–72.

Plato, *The Republic* (trans) Lee, D. (1956) (Harmondsworth: Penguin).

Popkin, R. and Stroll, A. (1969), *Philosophy Made Simple* (London: Heinemann).

Rachels, J. (1986), *The End of Life* (Oxford: Oxford University Press).

Raphael, D. D. (1981), *Moral Philosophy* (Oxford: Oxford University Press).

Raphael, D. D. (1990), *Problems of Political Philosophy*, 2nd ed. (London: Macmillan).

Rawls, J. (1971), *A Theory of Justice* (Oxford: Oxford University Press).

Robertson, G. (1993), 'Resuscitation and senility: a study of patients' opinions', *Journal of Medical Ethics*, 19, pp. 104–7.

Rowson, R. (1990), *An Introduction to Ethics for Nurses* (London: Scutari Press).

Russell, B. (1912), *The Problems of Philosophy* (Oxford: Oxford University Press).

Ross, P. (1994), *De-Privatising Morality* (Aldershot: Avebury).

Schecter, W. P. (1992), 'Surgical care of the HIV-infected patient', *Cambridge Quarterly of Healthcare Ethics*, 3, pp. 223–8.

Schon, D. A. (1987), *Educating the Reflective Practitioner* (San Francisco: Jossey-Bass).

Seedhouse, D. (1988), *Ethics the Heart of Health Care* (Chichester: John Wiley).

Singer, P. (1979), *Practical Ethics* (Cambridge: Cambridge University Press).

Singer, P. (ed.) (1986), *Applied Ethics* (Oxford: Oxford University Press).

Singer, P. (1993), *Practical Ethics*, 2nd ed. (Cambridge: Cambridge University Press).

Singer, P. (ed.) (1991), *A Companion to Ethics* (Oxford: Oxford University Press).

Sipes-Metzler, P. R. (1994), 'Oregon health plan: ration or reason?', *Journal of Medicine and Philosophy*, 19, pp. 305–14.

Smart, J. J. C. and Williams, B. (1973), *Utilitarianism For and Against* (Oxford: Clarendon Press).

Tadd, V. (1991), 'Where are the whistleblowers?', *Nursing Times*, 87 (1), pp. 42–4.

Thompson, I. E. , Melia, K. M. and Boyd, K. M. (1988), *Nursing Ethics* (London: Churchill Livingstone).

Tronto, J. (1987), 'Beyond gender difference', in Larrabee (ed.) (1993), pp. 240–57.

UKCC (1984), *Code of Professional Conduct* (London: UKCC).

UKCC (1989), *Exercising Accountability* (London: UKCC).

UKCC (1992), *Code of Professional Conduct* (London: UKCC).

Viens, D. C. (1990), 'AIDS and ethics', *California Nurse* (November), pp. 8–12.

Voluntary Euthanasia Society (1992), *The Last Right* (London: VES).

Williams, B. (1972), *Morality: an Introduction to Ethics* (Harmondsworth: Penguin).

Wolff, R. (1977), *Understanding Rawls* (Princeton: Princeton University Press).

Woods, S. and Edwards, S. D. (1989), 'Philosophy and health', *Journal of Advanced Nursing*, 14, pp. 661–4.

Wright, S. (1993), 'What makes a person?', *Nursing Times*, 89 (21), pp. 42–5.

Yarling, R. R. and McElmurry, B. J. (1983), 'Rethinking the nurse's role in "do not resuscitate" orders', *Advances in Nursing Science*, 5, pp. 1–12.

Index